95% OF ALL WOMEN HAVE SOME CELLULITE

But its causes and treatment are largely unknown in the U.S. However, in Europe, physicians have been analyzing cellulite for years.

Dr. Elisabeth Dancey, a British-born M.D., has spent time in Belgium studying cellulite removal and now brings you these proven techniques.

In easy-to-understand terms, she expains the complex circulatory system, how cells and body fat are nourished, how the body removes toxins from the cells, and what goes wrong to create cellulite.

A healthy diet and exercise program are not enough to eliminate cellulite. So how do you get rid of those ugly bumps and bulges?

Find out in *The Cellulite Solution*.

The
Cellulite
Solution

Dr. Elisabeth Dancey

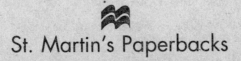

St. Martin's Paperbacks

First published in Great Britain in 1996 by Hodder & Stoughton
A division of Hodder Headline PLC

THE CELLULITE SOLUTION

Copyright © 1996 by Dr. Elisabeth Dancey.
Exercise illustrations by Sue Sharples; others by Rodney Paull.

Cover photograph by Hiroshi Hara.

ISBN: 0-312-96252-5

Printed in the United States of America

Hodder & Stoughton trade paperback edition published in 1996
St. Martin's Paperbacks edition/June 1997

10 9 8 7 6 5 4 3 2

To David, with love

ACKNOWLEDGMENTS

I would like to thank Jack, Barbara, Alexandra and Laura for their help, support and invaluable assistance in the preparation of this book.

CONTENTS

INTRODUCTION

Cellulite? Fat? Or what? Just exactly what do we mean when we use the term "cellulite"? What is it? How did we get it? How do we treat it?

Probably you are one of the 95 per cent of women who have, or think you have, cellulite. Quite possibly, you have tried various "treatments"—diets, exercise, creams, wraps, massages. You name it, you've tried it—*but* you *still* have cellulite. Why?

First, let's get one thing clear. It's not just "fat" women who suffer from cellulite. Even thin women are afflicted too. I've seen them in my surgery—we've all seen them. And not every "fat" woman gets cellulite, yet those who do may lose their "cellulite" when they lose their excess weight. So is it really cellulite or is it just fat?

Many women find that when they gain weight, they gain it on their lower body—the thighs, bottom and knees—the very area that is most commonly affected by cellulite. And when they lose weight, they lose it from their upper body. For some women, it seems almost impossible to gain weight on top or lose it from below. In fact, the harder they try, the more pear-shaped they seem to become. In some cases, exercise seems to make the legs chunkier and heavier, and some activities seem more prone to develop the legs than others. Why is it that the more exercise we do, the bigger our legs seem to get, and how might this be related to cellulite? I'll be giving you the answers to all these questions—and much, much more.

Thankfully, cellulite is now being accepted as a real medical condition rather than just a superficial beauty problem. By the time you have finished this book, you will not only understand why you suffer from it, but you should also be well on the way to getting rid of it.

We'll start by making a few observations. Then we will explain these, gradually, in simple scientific terms, so that you understand exactly how cellulite develops, spreads and how it responds to various treatments. You will also be able to appreciate why some of the methods you have tried have or haven't worked, and why some may even have made your condition worse.

Finally, men don't get cellulite—or do they? Although they do not sufer from "true" cellulite, as we'll discuss later in this book, men can have what is known as "dysmorphism" (footballer's legs) or cellulite-like fatty tissue on the tummy.

We all have our own personal experiences of cellulite, and our failures. And often we find that our experiences match everyone else's. So why don't we get any closer to resolving this problem?

Until recently, few doctors in Britain have acknowledged the existence of cellulite and, consequently, there has been little research, few hard facts and much nonsense written about the subject. On the Continent, however, GPs and hospital doctors are devoted to its study and treatment, and much time and money is spent on research. After all, they consider it a real health problem rather than just a mere inconvenience. Now, with a greater understanding and increased collaboration with our European colleagues, we can benefit from their knowledge, methods and products and put them into practice.

Getting rid of your cellulite will require certain changes to your lifestyle. Yet diet and exercise alone is not the answer. What you need is more information, commonsense advice and encouragement combined with simple self-help measures and recommendations on practical treatment methods. The aim of this book, therefore, is to show how, based on my knowledge and experience of treating cellulite both in Britain and overseas, it is possible to cure the symptoms and banish the problem for good.

HOW TO USE THIS BOOK

This book is divided into two parts. Part One deals with the basic principles, explaining just how and where cellulite forms and the factors that lead to its development. You will learn that there are a range of disorders that come under the general term of cellulite and a number of causes. In order to treat cellulite effectively, it is essential to understand which type of cellulite you have and what factors caused it since this will affect the type of treatment that is required.

Part Two deals with the various treatment methods and shows what steps you can take to get rid of your cellulite and prevent it from re-occurring. You will discover how best to treat yourself through diet, exercise and the use of creams, plant products, vegetable extracts and aromatherapy oils. The range of medical and other professional techniques is also explored to allow you, where necessary, to follow up with more intensive treatment and maximise your own self-help efforts.

As you read through this book you will come across certain scientific terms with which you may not already be familiar. Don't be alarmed. They are just names that we doctors use to describe parts of the body, disorders and treatments. If you're in any doubt, there is a glossary at the back of the book (see pages 180–197). These seemingly complex terms will be used over and over again and they will become second nature to you. As you progress through the book you will understand why it is important to include such detailed information. Most women are keen to know all they can about their bodies but, unfortunately, the real facts on cellulite are difficult to come by and many myths have been generated. My aim is to replace these myths with hard facts so that you can truly understand how cellulite develops and then get to grips with the treatment.

There may be a few surprises in store for you on the treatment side. Some treatments which you might never have imagined could help have been included, while others that you may have believed were useful have been omitted. This book is the fruit of research and my personal experience of treating cellulite throughout Europe, and I have included only those therapies and regimens that have been tested and proven to be successful. Others have not stood the test of time or medical scrutiny, or are simply not based on sound facts. You deserve the truth. Women are neither foolish nor frivolous consumers—we simply want to rid ourselves of an unpleasant, unnecessary and unsightly condition and we need all the help we can get. Here it is.

The
Cellulite
Solution

PART ONE:
THE BASIC PRINCIPLES

But isn't cellulite just fat? How many times have you heard that? And how many times have you been told all you need to do is take a bit more exercise, cut down on the fat in your diet and drink lots of water, and the cellulite will go? Probably too many times to remember! Let's be honest, you've started to take more exercise and improved your diet, but the cellulite still has not shifted. Why?

Cellulite is primarily a lifestyle problem. In recent years we have become more sedentary, and we are consuming ever greater quantities of processed foods or ready-made meals containing additives, artificial sweeteners, flavourings, colourings and other artificial products. Our way of life seems to be more stressful and we are exposed to a greater number of free radicals in the form of pollution, sunlight and smoking. Is it any wonder that our bodies suffer as a consequence?

Alarmingly, more and more girls are getting patches of cellulite at an early age, some as young as fourteen. The consumption of "junk foods," an early start to taking of the contraceptive pill, the decrease in exercise levels, particularly in the teenage years, earlier puberty and increased responsibility leading to extra stress all contribute to this.

All these factors ultimately cause damage to our bodies and are influential in the development of cellulite. To tackle cellulite, therefore, it is necessary to bring the body back into balance.

A whole industry has evolved to help us achieve this aim—creams, lotions, pills and potions. Each year appears a new breed of "miracle" cures and a never-ending supply of eager customers. We now have a vast array of treatments available to us, some useful and some of dubious worth. But these would not be possible were it not for the enormous development in medical techniques and investigations.

Through the availability of ultrasound, X-rays, thermal imaging and Doppler techniques, we are now able to study cellulite as a medical entity rather than dismiss it as a mere beauty problem. And in doing so, we have been able to discover that cellulite has a most definite start and end point and follows much the same course in all sufferers. Furthermore, we have been able to analyse the results of successful treatment—and if something can be successfully treated on a clinical level, it has to be a medical problem in the first place.

This section covers all the known causes of cellulite, but first it is important to get to grips with the basic principles if we are to fully understand how cellulite develops and then how best we can help ourselves. Read on, persevere, and you will be all the wiser after just a few more pages.

1

MORE THAN JUST FAT

Cellulite and fat are not the same

So what is the difference between cellulite and fat? Cellulite is, indeed, mostly fat, but it's not ordinary fatty tissue; it's fatty tissue that has been damaged as a result of certain malfunctions in the body's systems.

No matter how thin we are, we all have some fatty tissue just underneath the skin, and it is this fatty tissue that can develop into cellulite. This is probably the most important concept to remember. But in order to understand how and why this happens, first we need to know more about fat itself—how it is formed, why it's there and how we gain or lose it.

THE FACTS ABOUT FAT

To understand cellulite we need to know more about fat

A certain amount of fat in the diet is essential as it has several important functions. Most of the fat we eat is stored by the body until it is needed for energy—it's like filling up the freezer with food in case of future emergencies. In fact, the body tends to use, and prefers, sugar as an energy source. Sugars are easy to absorb and easy to burn to provide energy. However, very little sugar can be stored by the body and, as such, is kept as reserves in the liver as glycogen and used as a short-term energy store. When this store is full, any excess sugar is stored as fat.

So what happens to the fat we eat? This is absorbed in the small intestine and passes to the liver where some of it is used to make essential hormones, nerves, skin and other body structures. Any excess is sent over to the fatty tissues via the blood and stored in the fat cells.

Fat is a wonderful insulating tissue. It allows us to retain our body heat and protects delicate organs and structures such as the kidneys, heart, liver and lungs from damage. Fat just under the skin gives us protection from knocks and bumps as well as protecting our bony protuberances from the damage of prolonged pressure, for instance by cushioning the bones of the bottom on which we sit. Furthermore, chemicals, pesticides and other unwanted products contained in the food and water we consume are stored in the body's fat, and this helps protect the more important tissues from their adverse effects. Fat is also important for the absorption of the fat-soluble vitamins A, D, E and K.

However, excess fat in the diet can be harmful and most of us consume far too much. We are all only too aware of the problems of heart disease and its association with fat intake. In an ideal world, our fat intake would be matched to our needs—the fat would be deposited where it was needed in the body and not where it could do us harm. But, of course, life is not so simple and there are many interacting factors that affect our body fat distribution.

BODY FAT DISTRIBUTION

All fat is not equal

Exactly where we store our body fat depends on our sex, our genetic make-up, our lifestyle and our hormone balance. Most men are apple-shaped, tending to store their fat around the tummy, heart and intestines, whilst women tend to be pear-shaped, storing fat on the bottom, hips and thighs.

Excess fat is stored in fat cells in the fatty tissue. We lay down fat cells during childhood and adolescence, and once these fat cells have been laid down they cannot normally be removed. All we can do is shrink them, but we can't reduce their number. There are certain factors that influence how and where body fat is stored and removed, so let's have a look at some of these.

THE STORAGE AND REMOVAL OF FAT

Located on the surface of each fat cell are microscopic structures known as receptors, and it is these receptors that control the storage and removal of fat. Think of them as little doors that open and close, responding to certain chemical messengers in the body by either letting fat in or out of the fat cells.

Research has shown that there are several types of receptors; some enable the storage of fat and others enable its removal. The ones that control the *storage* of fat in the fat cells are known as *alpha-2* receptors, and these are stimulated by insulin released when there is excess fat in the bloodstream, for instance after a meal. Sugar in excess can also be transformed into fat and stored via the alpha-2 receptors in the same way.

Receptors that control the *release* of fat from the fat cells back into the bloodstream are known as *beta* receptors. These are stimulated by the hormones thyroxine and adrenaline and other naturally occurring substances.

If we want to encourage the removal of fat we need to know exactly which chemicals and drugs will mimic the effect of the body's natural hormones and thus trick the beta receptors into "opening up" and releasing fat.

In fact, there are several compounds and medicines which will do just that. Caffeine, aminophylline (an asthma drug), silicium, cobalt, zinc and manganese in minute quantities can all stimulate the fat-releasing beta receptors, but we need to know how best to take them in order to achieve the desired results. For instance, caffeine taken orally in small doses increases the metabolic rate (the rate at which we burn calories), but if taken in too high doses, it causes the blood vessels to narrow, thus restricting the flow of blood—an unwanted effect when treating cellulite. When applied directly to the skin, however, caffeine permeates it easily to stimulate the fat-releasing beta receptors.

Similarly, the drug aminophylline, when applied locally, penetrates the skin to stimulate the beta receptors, but if taken by mouth it mainly affects the lung tissue, and the fat cells remain untouched.

The release of fat is also governed by the amount of blood that passes through the tissues. A rich blood supply will ensure a rapid release of fat, thereby allowing a greater volume of fat to be removed from the fat cells. Therefore, the better and more plentiful the blood supply through the tissues, the faster the fat can be mobilised when necessary. Cellulite tissue, as we will discover, has a very poor blood supply.

FAT CELLS AND WEIGHT GAIN

The distribution of fat-storing and fat-releasing receptors around the body influences where we store fat. Why is it that women seem to carry most of their weight on the bottom, hips, thighs and inner knees, yet when they try to lose weight, it seems to come off the top first—the chest, arms and face and neck?

There's no doubt that when women gain weight they tend to gain it on the lower body, and when they lose weight it seems to fall off the upper body but remains stubbornly attached to the bottom, legs and thighs. In fact, the more they continue to diet, the more the weight seems to disappear from the top, and then when they stop dieting and regain the weight, the bigger the bottom and thighs become. And the more they repeat this lose-gain-lose-gain cycle, the more pear-shaped they become. Unfair, or just a fact of life?

The reason for this is that the fat cells in the bottom, thighs and the inner area of the knees—the most common cellulite trouble spots—seem to respond in a different way to fat consumed in the diet than fat cells elsewhere in the body.

Research has shown that in most women the fat cells around the bottom, thighs and knees have a greater proportion of fat-storing alpha-2 receptors and a lesser proportion of fat-releasing beta receptors than fat cells elsewhere in the body. Further research has enabled us to quantify this difference: in the bottom, thighs and knees there are approximately six fat-storing receptors for every fat-releasing receptor. The situation is exactly the reverse on the upper body.

The fat cells in these cellulite-prone areas are therefore more avid, more hungry for fat and, hence, more ready to store fat than fat cells elsewhere in the body. Yet, their capacity to release fat is reduced by a factor of six. In real terms, this means that if we were to gain 7kg of fat, six of these would be gained on the bottom, hips and thighs and only 1kg on the upper body. Conversely, if we lost 7kg, only 1kg would come off the lower body and the other 6kg from the upper body. The more this lose-gain cycle is continued, the more this pattern is repeated. This is why the fluctuation of weight caused by repeated dieting—the yo-yo effect—will change the pattern of fat distribution and, hence, body shape.

Interestingly enough, a new fat-storing receptor has just been discovered in men. Some men have a greater proportion of fat-storing receptors around the tummy and intestines—the typical fat-storage site for men—than elsewhere in the body. So this does seem to confirm that the pattern of fat storage is determined by genetics and sex. This may indicate a hormonal influence or suggest that the fat-storage gene only works in the presence of either of the sex chromosomes.

- Some fat is essential for the body to function efficiently.
- Excess fat is stored in fat cells in the fatty tissue.

- Alpha-2 receptors on the cell surface allow the deposition of fat in the fat cell.
- Beta receptors on the cell surface allow the release of fat from the fat cell.
- Fat cells on the bottom, thighs and knees have six times more fat-storing alpha-2 receptors than fat-releasing beta receptors.
- Fat cells on the upper body have six times more fat-releasing beta receptors than fat-storing alpha-2 receptors.
- Fat is preferentially stored on the lower body and released from the upper body.
- A rich and plentiful blood supply through fatty tissue is necessary for the mobilisation of fat.

2

A HEALTHY BLOOD SUPPLY

A malfunction in the blood supply system is a key element in the development of cellulite

Blood is literally the life force of the body, and maintaining a rich and plentiful blood supply to the fatty tissues is crucial in the prevention of cellulite. Blood consists of a mixture of red blood cells that carry oxygen, white blood cells that fend off disease, platelets that help the blood to clot when needed and plasma, a protein-rich fluid that carries nutrients, proteins, hormones, waste substances and water.

BLOOD SUPPLY TO THE TISSUES

How the cells are nourished

All tissue is made up of cells—Nature's building blocks. These are stacked together and held in place by fibrous tissue—Nature's cement. All cells have a job to do and for this they need a constant supply of oxygen and nutrients, which are carried in the blood.

The red blood cells are filled with oxygen (oxygenated) from the lungs and then blood is pumped around the body by the heart; first the oxygenated blood passes through large arteries to reach all parts of the body. Arteries are strong muscular vessels which can pulsate, and it is this pulsating action which helps the blood to flow through the tissues.

When the arteries finally reach their destination, the tissues, they branch off into small arterioles and then into fine capillaries that mingle in between the individual cells. Once amongst the cells, fluid from the blood leaves the capillaries to bathe the cells in oxygen and nutrients. These small capillaries which supply oxygenated blood to the tissues are known as the microcirculation.

Oxygen and nutrients are then used by the cells to provide energy for vital growth, repair and division. This process is known as respiration. It's rather like an engine burning petrol to create energy. The waste products of this process—the exhaust of our engine if you like—are water, carbon dioxide, lactic acid and toxins. Just as the exhaust fumes need to be expelled from the engine, the lactic acid and toxins need to be removed from the tissues, otherwise they will cause damage. These are therefore returned to the blood in the veins where they are neutralised to form non-toxic substances such as carbon dioxide and water.

The blood, once it has passed through the tissues, is now devoid of oxygen and is known as deoxygenated blood. It looks more purple than red, and this is invariably the blood you see when you cut yourself. The deoxygenated blood now has to be returned to the heart via the veins. First, it flows through tiny capillaries which join up into small veins (venules) which unite and form bigger veins on their way back to the heart.

Unlike the arteries, the veins and lymph vessels do not have any muscles within their walls and rely on three separate mechanisms to return the blood and fluid to the general circulation. These three mechanisms are extremely relevant when we come to look at both the development and treatment of cellulite.

RETURN OF BLOOD AND FLUID FROM THE LEGS

The veins and lymph vessels return blood and fluid to the circulation by means of three mechanisms

CONTRACTION OF THE SURROUNDING LEG MUSCLES

The blood vessels in the legs are surrounded by muscles. When these muscles contract they exert a pressure on the veins and lymph vessels which forces blood and lymph back towards the heart. The presence of one-way valves in the veins prevents the back flow of blood. Probably the most important muscles involved in this mechanism are the calf muscles.

Fluid from within the blood passes out through the walls of the capillaries to seep amongst the tissues. The fluid is now known as tissue fluid. The fluid seeps through the tissues, nourishing them and removing some of the toxic waste products. Some of the tissue fluid is collected by the veins, the rest is removed from the tissues by the lymph vessels. Similar to the veins, these are delicate vessels that intertwine amongst the tissues, removing excess fluid. The fluid is now known as lymph. The lymph vessels join up to form larger and larger vessels, eventually returning the lymph to the general circulation via connections to the large veins at the base of the neck.

THE PLANTAR RETURN REFLEX

There is an interesting, but often poorly appreciated, reflex area in the sole of the foot which also stimulates the return of lymph. The plantar fascia (the fibrous tissue running between the heel of the foot and the base of the toes) contains numerous receptors which, when stimulated, encourage the return of lymph. This reflex is often used, albeit subconsciously, by people such as policemen and soldiers who may have to stand motionless for hours at a time. Gentle movement of the foot to stretch and stimulate the plantar fascia will ensure that they do not collapse from faintness or suffer from varicose veins! Rocking onto tiptoe to bring the calf muscles into play will further improve the venous and lymphatic return. Dancers, particularly ballroom dancers, who use the sole of the foot a lot in their movements, have fine legs because they are constantly stimulating their plantar return reflex and ensuring a rapid return of lymph to the heart.

THE THORACO-ABDOMINAL PUMP

The return of lymph and venous blood is also aided by what is known as the thoraco-abdominal pump. When the diaphragm contracts in breathing, it descends and creates a negative pressure in the thorax (chest)—like a pulling or sucking action. This negative pressure draws up blood and lymph from the abdomen into the thorax, ready for return to the heart. At the same time, the descent of the diaphragm pushes on the abdominal cavity and causes an increase in pressure which also pushes the blood and lymph into the thorax. The result is a flow of lymph and venous blood from the legs and surrounding areas to the centre of the body. The back and side walls of the abdomen have rigid bony and muscular supports. The front wall of the abdomen is formed by the abdominal muscles, which should be strong but all too often are flabby. It is the strength of these tummy muscles that allow the thoraco-abdominal pump to work. If the tummy muscles are flabby, the diaphragm will move downwards in inspiration (breathing in), but the tummy will sag and no pressure will be generated to "push" blood and lymph into the thorax. Strong tummy muscles will provide a resistance against the descending diaphragm and allow sufficient pressure to be generated in the abdomen to help the return of fluid.

It is important that the arteries, veins and lymph vessels are working properly to keep the fatty tissue nourished and to remove waste products and tissue fluid. As we shall see later, it is a breakdown in one or more of these systems that allows cellulite to take hold.

- Blood carries oxygen and nutrients through the arteries to the cells (blood supply).
- Deoxygenated blood, containing carbon dioxide and toxins, returns to the lungs via the veins (venous return).
- Lymph fluid from the tissues trickles into the lymphatic system to be returned to the blood (lymphatic return).
- Venous blood and lymph are returned to the circulation via three mechanisms:
  - the contraction of the surrounding muscles
  - the stimulation of the plantar return reflex
  - the action of the thoraco-abdominal pump.

3

FAT TO CELLULITE—HOW IT HAPPENS

So, when does fat become cellulite? What controls it? And, more importantly, how can we influence it?

We now know that in order for the cells and tissues to function properly they need an efficient blood transport and waste-removal system. This means a rich supply of blood to carry oxygen and nutrients, a good venous system to remove the carbon dioxide and toxins, and a good lymphatic drainage system to remove the tissue fluid (lymph).

The use of sophisticated scientific techniques such as Doppler, ultrasound, lymphangiography and echography has enabled us to discover exactly what happens in the tissues as they develop cellulite. Such techniques have commonly been used both in the diagnosis and treatment of circulatory disorders such as leg ulcers, poor circulation and fluid retention. On the Continent, they have been used to study cellulite and have revealed a wealth of information that helps us to understand how cellulite develops and, more importantly, how we can intervene in order to treat it.

Even more refined techniques used only in research laboratories have allowed us to investigate exactly how the cells react under certain conditions, and these techniques have given us an enormous insight into the functioning of fat cells and other cells that control and regulate the subcutaneous tissue—the fatty tissue just underneath the skin, which is where cellulite develops.

We now know that the distribution of fat-storing and fat-releasing receptors on the cell surface affects where we store fat on our bodies and that the pattern of fat storage is related to the sex of the individual. I'm afraid, where Nature is concerned, sex discrimination knows no bounds! Men have a higher proportion of fat-storing receptors around the tummy and intestines, whilst women have a greater proportion on the bottom, thighs and knees. This is probably due to hormones or genetics, or more likely an interaction of both. We already know that women can react adversely to certain hormones, such as those in the contraceptive pill, by gaining weight.

In women, the tendency to gain weight on the lower body and to lose it from the upper body will not in itself lead to cellulite; it will just exaggerate their existing pear shape. However, since cellulite develops in fatty tissue, it stands to reason it will tend to occur in the very areas that contain most fat which, in this case, means the bottom, thighs and knees.

Cellulite occurs when fatty tissue is damaged, so let's look at what causes this. Although there are three main factors that are involved, the essential thing to understand is that all three factors interact with each other. Insufficient blood supply via the microcirculation, insufficient clearance of tissue fluid by the veins and the lymphatic system can eventually lead to cellulite. Remember that cellulite develops in fatty tissue; it is the amount of fatty tissue affected that determines the amount of cellulite that appears on the body. Although certain genetic factors may come into play, cellulite is largely a lifestyle problem. There are many underlying causes that can result in excess fat storage, damage to the microcirculation or a disturbance in the venous and lymphatic system. All the precipitating factors that can ultimately lead to cellulite will be discussed in Chapter 5.

WHAT CAUSES TISSUE DAMAGE?

MICROCIRCULATION

Damage to the microcirculation will lead to cellulite

As we saw in the previous chapter, arteries carrying oxygen and nutrient-rich blood divide into smaller and smaller vessels until they become capillaries. At the point where these tiny capillaries surround the cells of the tissue, the oxygen and nutrients are released. This is what we call the microcirculation.

Damage to the microcirculation means that oxygen and nutrients cannot reach the tissues in the amounts needed for normal cell metabolism, which results in a certain degree of tissue starvation and a build-up of waste products and toxins in this area. In the short term, there are no ill consequences. We have all experienced this, for instance in winter when our hands get really cold and turn blue as the amount of blood entering the hands decreases. The reason for this is that the arteries sense that the temperature is very low and therefore limit the amount of blood going into the hands—non-vital parts of the body. This is an entirely normal reaction. What happens is that the blood vessels in the arms constrict (narrow) to prevent too much warm blood reaching a very cold surface which would result in a loss of essential body heat. The hands feel cold and turn blue—a sign that there is a build-up of carbon dioxide in the blood. But as well as carbon dioxide, there are also toxins which need a good supply of oxygen in order to be neutralised.

As soon as we come in from the cold and the risk of losing body heat is past, the arteries sense the increase in heat, so they open up again and the hands warm up once more as the blood supply returns. However, the arteries do not just open up to the same width as before but even wider so that a good supply of oxygen floods into the tissues to neutralise the toxins as rapidly as possible. The hands start to throb and feel very warm, almost painful for a while. The medical term for this is reactive hyperaemia and it is a totally normal occurrence. It is the body's way of rapidly removing waste products and toxins that would otherwise damage tissue. After a few minutes, the redness and throbbing settle down and the hands return to their normal colour. The toxins have been completely removed.

However, if the arteries were to remain "shut down" so that there was not the capacity for extra blood to flow into the tissues after exposure to the cold, then a very different situation would arise. An insufficient supply of oxygen and nutrients to the tissues and, hence, insufficient neutralisation of toxins, would result in tissue damage. This is what happens in the formation of cellulite tissue—but in this instance it is factors other than exposure to the cold that stimulate a shut-down of the arteries.

Cellulite tissue, as we shall discover later, has a poor circulation. The relative lack of oxygen and nutrients leads to a build-up of toxic waste products called metabolites. These toxic metabolites not only cause damage to the existing tissue but also affect the way that new tissue-building takes place.

Within the tissues themselves are fibre-making cells known as fibroblasts. These fibroblasts make tiny fibres that form a supporting meshwork around the fat cells to bind the whole structure together, gently but firmly—like tissue cement. However, if the fibroblasts are deprived of oxygen and nourishment, instead of making fine fibres they make thick knots of mucopolysaccharides—heavy fibres that surround and envelop the fat cells. It is the build-up of these thick fibres that is one of the reasons for that familiar "tethering" effect seen in cellulite.

In advanced cases of cellulite a few arteries remain amongst the cellulite tissue that are not too damaged by the cellulite-forming process. These arteries are still able to respond to the huge amount of metabolic toxins that have accumulated amongst the cells. They therefore open up as wide as possible to allow in oxygen-rich blood to neutralise the toxins. This results in islands of warm tissue amongst a sea of cold cellulite tissue, which is quite obvious to the touch. Anyone who has cellulite will no doubt recognise some of these familiar symptoms—from the early signs to later evidence of advanced cellulite.

The rate at which fat is metabolised—that is, freed from fatty tissue—depends upon the circulation of oxygen and nutrients through it as well as the number of fat-releasing receptors in that particular area. So fatty tissue that has a rich blood supply will easily be burnt up when the body calls upon that fat for energy. However, if the microcirculation is disturbed, insufficient blood reaches the tissues and the fat simply cannot be used up. The result is a stubborn mass of unavailable fat.

- Lack of oxygen in the tissues causes a build-up of toxic waste products known as metabolites.
- Toxic metabolites cause damage to tissue.
- Poor oxygenation of the tissues allows thick, tethering cellulite fibres to develop around the fat cells.
- Poor blood supply prevents the removal of fat from fatty tissue.

VEINS

Damage to the veins also leads to cellulite

The removal of blood through the veins (venous drainage) also plays an important role in maintaining the health of fatty tissue.

Blood, which is now carrying carbon dioxide and waste products, is cleared from the tissues by the capillaries, which reunite and form veins. The veins eventually neutralise their toxic waste products and discharge their carbon dioxide in the lungs.

However, if the flow of blood in the veins slows down, this creates a certain back-pressure in the system which is transmitted back through the veins and eventually into the tissues. It's like a traffic jam where a blockage at one end of the road will quickly lead to a build-up of traffic and exhaust, and will disrupt the flow from behind. Likewise, a blockage in the veins ultimately leads to a build-up of toxic metabolites in the tissues which causes damage to both the tissues and walls of the veins, resulting in localised inflammation. Inflammation of the veins causes their walls to weaken and to release further, more potent substances, including arachidonic acid. Arachidonic acid and other substances in turn cause more inflammatory damage, resulting in painful, swollen tissues.

When the vein walls are sufficiently weakened, blood leaks out into the tissues, causing further pain and inflammation. Some of these changes are microscopic, others are visible to the naked eye. In some instances, the veins become massively enlarged resulting in varicose veins. Some veins merely swell, but the smaller veins just break, releasing blood into the surrounding tissues and causing bruising and discolouration.

Varicose veins, swollen veins and broken veins all stem from increased pressure in the venous system and all can lead to the development of cellulite. When the veins have reached this advanced stage of damage, they can no longer remove blood from the tissues and so the back-pressure on the tissues is further increased. Thus, a vicious cycle is created: increased pressure leads to more damage to the veins, and more damage to the veins leads to more pressure—and more cellulite.

- A build-up of toxic metabolites in the veins causes the release of arachidonic acid and other tissue-damaging substances.
- Arachidonic acid and other waste products cause damage to the vein walls, making them leaky.
- Leaky veins allow blood and tissue fluid to seep into the tissues and cause further damage.
- Increased venous pressure causes varicose, swollen and broken veins.
- Varicose, swollen and broken veins cause cellulite.

LYMPHATIC DRAINAGE

Poor lymphatic drainage almost always causes cellulite

Waste-laden fluid in the tissues must be removed via the lymphatic drainage system in order to maintain healthy cells. The importance of the lymphatic system was first appreciated by an Austrian doctor, Dr. Emil Vodder, and his wife in the early 1930s, to whom we still owe much of our knowledge and understanding today. One of the most prominent features of the lymphatic system is its fragility, and Dr. Vodder was the first to stress the need to respect its delicate anatomy. It is only years later that we have been able to appreciate the value of his work.

In a recent study at Brussels University, lymphangiograms (a medical investigation which determines the structure and flow of the lymph system) were performed on all women who presented themselves at the university's cellulite clinic. The results showed that the lymphatic system was deficient in all clients with cellulite. Lymphangiograms can be quite painful, and it is not necessary to perform them routinely on all clients, but the above study serves to show that the problem of a deficient lymphatic system must be addressed if cellulite is to be dealt with effectively.

Lymph is the fluid that escapes from the blood, quite naturally, and supplies the cells with oxygen and nutrients. Once it has done its job, lymph, now filled with toxins, is cleared from the tissues by the veins or the lymph vessels. However, lymph vessels are extremely fragile and can easily rupture or become squashed by outside pressure, both of which can disrupt the flow of lymph. If the flow is disrupted, the pressure within the tissues increases and creates a backlog of lymph.

Lymph fluid is rich in protein, rather like jelly, and when it flows freely, it poses no problems. However, if the flow slows down, the fluid sets just like jelly. The proteins separate out of the lymph and congeal, forming thick fibres. The fluid becomes thicker and the flow slows down further. Another vicious circle.

Over time, these fibres are thickened further by the addition of more protein or by the action of fibroblasts, the fibre-making cells in the tissues. Remember that when the fibroblasts are deprived of oxygen and nutrients, they make abnormal, thick fibres. Now they have thick, protein-rich lymph fibres to use as a base on which to spin their own thick fibres. You can see how the problem is compounded and, by now, you can begin to appreciate the interactive role of the microcirculation, the venous and lymphatic drainage in the development of cellulite.

Lymph fibres, thickened by the action of the fibroblasts, become heavy, abnormal and form a honeycomb around the fat cells which accounts for that familiar tethering effect seen in cellulite. Fluid becomes trapped between the cells and the fibres, making the tissue waterlogged, firm to the touch and further increasing the tissue pressure. The increased tissue pressure prevents blood flowing freely through the tissues. Consequently, the tissues become a path of high resistance so that the blood now tends to go round rather than through it—like traffic avoiding the congested city centre, preferring to take the free-flowing ringroad. The resulting fat and fluid honeycomb is what creates the lumpy, irregular, tethered, tender area of fatty tissue that we recognise as cellulite.

In severe cases, the fibres encircling the fat and fluid can virtually isolate huge lumps, forming ever larger honeycombs known as "steatomes." These steatomes protrude from the normal silhouette of the body and result in those characteristic lumps and bumps on the surface of the skin.

Since the blood flow has now been re-routed around rather than through the cellulite tissue, the cells, in particular the fibroblasts, are deprived of essential oxygen and nutrients. Fat is unable to be removed from the fat cells and remains a virtual prisoner, trapped inside a thick bag of fibres.

- Lymph vessels are very fragile.
- Lymph fluid contains proteins, which can separate out of the fluid and set like jelly if the flow of lymph is disrupted.
- Once it sets, lymph fluid forms thick, tethering fibres, which are made even thicker by the action of fibroblasts.
- The fibres arrange themselves around the fat cells and may ultimately form "steatomes."

THE STEP-BY-STEP DEVELOPMENT OF CELLULITE

Cellulite develops in stages over a period of time

As we have seen, there are three chief factors that lead to the development of cellulite: damage to the microcirculation, venous drainage or lymphatic drainage. Since all these factors are interdependent, what tends to happen is that once the precipitating factor has taken hold, a whole chain reaction is set in motion whereby all three factors will ultimately become involved. Thus, for instance, what may start as a problem with the microcirculation will eventually cause disruption to the veins and lymphatic system. So, although in theory there are only three main origins of cellulite, in practice there is always some degree of overlap, and the overlap becomes greater as the condition progresses.

The areas of the body that are affected by cellulite depend on the degree of disruption to the microcirculatory, venous or lymphatic systems. The sheer volume of cellulite in a specific area, however, depends on the amount of fat stored in the fat cells in the cellulite tissue.

Figure 1 illustrates normal subcutaneous (fatty) tissue with a good blood supply giving oxygen and nutrients to the tissues. Fluid released by the capillaries to nourish the tissue is removed by the veins and lymph vessels and little or no fluid gathers between the cells. Fibroblasts that produce fibres are healthy and make normal fibres to support the tissue.

Cellulite tissue, however, illustrated in Figure 2, has a poor blood supply due to damage to the microcirculation. The fibroblasts are therefore starved of oxygen and vital nutrients and the veins and lymph vessels are unable to drain the tissues effectively. Fluid builds up in between the cells of the tissues and the protein within the fluid begins to settle out to form thick, inelastic fibres between the fat cells. The now unhealthy fibroblasts fail to remove the abnormal protein fibres. Pressure within the tissue increases and the tissue feels hard, tender and lumpy. The blood cannot pass through the rigid, tense tissue and so flows around rather than through it. The consequent lack of blood supply makes the situation worse, creating a vicious circle.

Cellulite does not appear overnight and, likewise, cannot be cured overnight. However, the severity of the cellulite and the length of time it has been established can affect the type of treatment that is required.

We know what happens on the inside of the body when cellulite takes hold, so let's link this to what we can see on the outside.

No matter how much cellulite we have or wherever it appears on the body, once it has started, it progresses in much the same way as all three factors come into play.

STAGE ONE

The first thing that happens is a general slowing down in the flow of blood through the microcirculation, the venous or lymphatic drainage.

A slowing down of the microcirculation means that the blood supply to the tissues is limited and the tissues will be more susceptible to invasion by cellulite, although at this stage there will be no visible signs. The only hint of early cellulite is that cuts or bruises may take longer than usual to heal.

A slowing down of the venous drainage results in a slight degree of fluid retention in the tissues. The blood flow in the smaller veins and capillaries comes almost to a standstill. Damaging substances such as arachidonic acid are released which irritate the walls of these small vessels, causing them to become inflamed.

A slowing down of the lymphatic drainage again results in fluid retention; lymph fluid begins to build up in the tissues and some

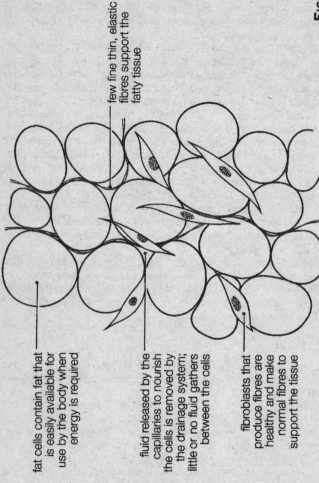

few fine thin, elastic fibres support the fatty tissue

fat cells contain fat that is easily available for use by the body when energy is required

fluid released by the capillaries to nourish the cells is removed by the drainage system; little or no fluid gathers between the cells

fibroblasts that produce fibres are healthy and make normal fibres to support the tissue

FIGURE 1

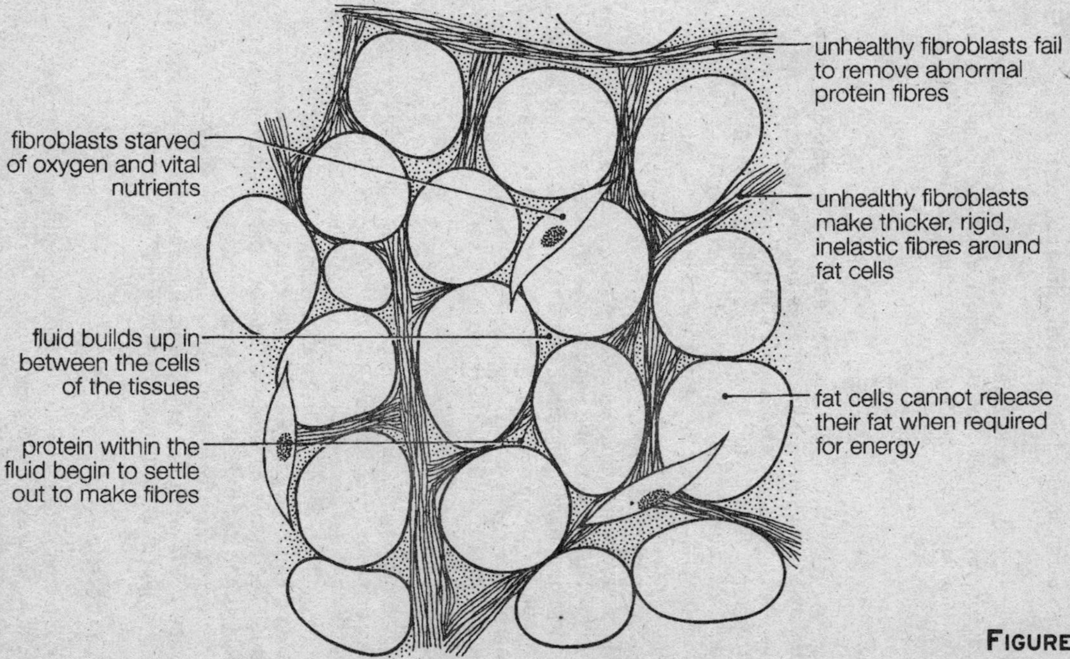

unhealthy fibroblasts fail to remove abnormal protein fibres

unhealthy fibroblasts make thicker, rigid, inelastic fibres around fat cells

fat cells cannot release their fat when required for energy

fibroblasts starved of oxygen and vital nutrients

fluid builds up in between the cells of the tissues

protein within the fluid begin to settle out to make fibres

FIGURE 2

protein may separate out from the fluid and set to form very fine fibres.

All the above changes are microscopic and not yet visible to the human eye. Nevertheless, the damage has set in and a slowing down in any of these systems will ultimately lead to a disruption in all three.

STAGE TWO

Once the chain has set in motion and the flow of blood has been disrupted, the veins and capillaries are now weakened. Just as a dam with weak walls will finally collapse under the pressure of the rising tide, likewise the veins and capillaries break down under the pressure from the backlog of blood. Blood and fluid now seep out amongst the tissues, increasing the tissue pressure and restricting the blood circulation and drainage processes still further.

You may notice broken veins and tiny areas of discolouration of the skin. If you were to squeeze the skin, it would feel thicker than normal, quite tender and painful, with a tendency to bruise easily. These are probably the first noticeable signs of cellulite and these symptoms may remain for some time before any further developments take place. At this stage, however, there is no overt swelling and no change in the temperature of the skin.

STAGE THREE

After a few weeks or months of fluid build-up within the tissues, the demands placed on the tiny lymph vessels far outstrip their ability to drain the tissues. In any case, the lymph vessels will have already been slightly damaged and possibly squashed by the increasing tissue pressure. Fluid retention is now a permanent feature. The tissues become swollen and thicker and begin to push against the hair follicles and sweat glands.

You will now be able to see obvious signs of swelling in the skin. The swollen skin starts to push against the hair follicles and sweat glands creating that characteristic "orange-peel" look.

STAGE FOUR

The lymph fluid is now at a virtual standstill, and this causes protein to separate out of the fluid and congeal into fibres. These fibres are made thicker by the action of fibroblasts deprived of oxygen and nutrients. The fibres form a meshwork around the fat cells, trapping fluid and creating the coarser tethering effect often referred to as "mattress skin."

Fluid retention leads to waterlogged tissues, which press on the microcirculation creating an area of high resistance. Blood chooses to bypass the congested area rather than flow through it. The lack of blood supply to the affected area causes the skin to feel quite cold to the touch.

Venous drainage and clearance of toxins and waste products is now compromised. The result is the vessels are easily broken, leading to bruises that heal very slowly.

STAGE FIVE

Increasing pressure within the tissues has now re-routed the flow of blood around the cellulite tissue rather than through it. The areas where the blood now flows are forced to respond to the presence of metabolic toxins nearby by opening up and allowing huge amounts of blood to pass through the affected area, forming hot islands amongst otherwise cold cellulite tissue.

STAGE SIX

Fibres continue to be formed around the fat cells in the affected area. Fat cannot be removed from the cells because of the poor blood supply. However, fat continues to be stored in the fat cells because of the preponderance of fat-storing receptors on the surface of the cells. So the fat increases, the fibres get thicker and thicker and increase in number, forming huge honeycombs of fat, fluid and fibre, known as steatomes.

Steatomes disfigure the silhouette of the body, forming bulky, unattractive lumps and bumps on the surface of the skin. The presence of steatomes is a pretty good indication that the cellulite is well established and suggests that the cellulite process has run its full course.

4

OTHER CELLULITE-PRONE AREAS

Cellulite may also present itself on the tummy, neck and arms

The most common cellulite trouble spots for women are the bottom, thighs and knees and, up till now, this is the type of cellulite we have been talking about. But cellulite can also appear on the tummy, the nape of the neck and the backs of the arms. And yes, men can suffer too!

ON THE TUMMY

Digestive problems can result in cellulite tissue on the tummy

The tummy, or abdomen, is a common site for the deposition of fat. Just about all of us at some time or other have complained at the state of our tummies and resolved to do something about it. Sure enough, this fat can be remarkably stubborn and extremely resistant to our attempts to shift it. The fat cells in this area often contain a large proportion of fat-storing receptors and a relatively small number of fat-releasing receptors on their surface. But this does not necessarily lead to cellulite. In most cases, it's pure fat and what is needed is a good weight-reducing diet and exercise programme—and an enormous supply of willpower! Some of the treatment techniques in Part Two of this book will also be invaluable in helping remove this obstinate layer of fat.

However, some people do suffer from cellulite on the tummy. But how can you tell whether it's normal fat or cellulite? Quite simply, cellulite will exhibit all the signs that we have discussed in the last chapter. There will be areas of dimpling, areas that are tender to the touch and areas that show signs of tethering. If you recognise these familiar symptoms, you can be sure it's cellulite.

Interestingly, however, the cause of abdominal cellulite is slightly different to the cause of cellulite on the lower body. So let me stretch your mind a little further. It's been stretched enough so far with facts and principles so it should be getting used to it by now!

According to acupuncturists, osteopaths and mesotherapists, all of whom use local skin injection or manipulation techniques, the area of skin between the ribcage and pubic bone is "connected" to the underlying digestive organs via a series of nerves. This means that any disorder in the liver, gall bladder, stomach and small and large intestines will manifest itself on certain areas of the skin on the abdomen, usually in the form of tenderness due to fluid retention in the underlying tissues. Dysfunctions such as a lazy, congested liver, gall bladder spasm or irritable bowel can be successfully diagnosed in this way and treated by injections, manipulation or massage to the appropriate area. However, none of the aforementioned practitioners would attempt to treat a severe problem which required medical or surgical intervention and, in any case, the signs on the skin would be far too confusing and unreliable for an accurate diagnosis.

A problem with an underlying organ is often one of inflammation. So, if a particular organ were slightly swollen or painful, the area of skin that referred to that organ would also show similar symptoms. For instance, if the large intestine were a little swollen, the skin on the abdomen that referred to the large intestine would also be swollen. Inflammation causes fluid retention in the fatty tissues and, here, we have stage one in the development of cellulite.

Very often people with cellulite have problems with digestion such as irritable bowel, constipation, or liver congestion or spasm. It is important that these conditions are treated, otherwise they will simply continue to "feed" the cellulite tissue on the tummy.

Stress, like disorders of the digestive organs, can manifest itself on the skin. Constant stress will deposit cellulite on the upper part of the tummy—just underneath the ribcage but well above the belly button.

As both men and women can suffer from digestive problems and stress, both are equally susceptible to suffering from cellulite on the tummy.

ON THE NECK

Constant stress can result in cellulite on the neck

Stress also shows itself on the nape of the neck and is almost always associated with neck, shoulder and arm pain. Over time, this leads to the development of the characteristic "Dowager's hump"—a fatty, cellulite-ridden lump on the back of the neck.

The reason for this is that sustained stress over a period of years causes the neck and shoulder muscles to pull on the vertebrae (the bones of the spine), eventually forcing them out of alignment and squashing the nerves in the neck and shoulders. This results in pain and localised inflammation. Again, inflammation causes fluid retention, which is translated onto the skin. And once more we have the first stage of cellulite.

ON THE UPPER ARMS

A disruption in the venous drainage system can cause cellulite on the upper arms

The upper arms are sometimes affected by cellulite, and such cellulite tends only to come on in later life. The effects can be particularly unpleasant, as it causes the arms to look heavy and the sleeves of clothing to feel uncomfortably tight. Cellulite on the upper arms is almost always caused by a problem with the venous drainage of the tissues and will almost inevitably be associated with cellulite elsewhere on the body, mostly on the legs. Other symptoms of venous disturbance are invariably present, such as broken veins, heavy legs and fluid retention.

DYSMORPHISM

Disturbance to the microcirculation and venous drainage can result in dysmorphism, commonly known as "footballer's legs"

There is an extremely common variation of cellulite that occurs in both men and women. Dysmorphism—or footballer's legs, as it is commonly called in the UK—is a cellulite condition that affects only the fronts of the thighs.

Dysmorphism arises out of a disturbance in the microcirculation and venous drainage in the fatty tissue on the front of the thighs. Although the general circulation and venous drainage of the leg muscles, in particular the front thigh muscles, are excellent, the circulation to and drainage from the overlying tissue is poor. Thus, when any muscular activity involving the legs is performed, blood enters the legs to supply the muscles with oxygen. The influx of blood overstretches the venous and lymphatic drainage of the legs, particularly in the subcutaneous tissue. Fluid therefore builds up and the tissue becomes swollen, thus setting the scene for the development of cellulite.

Thereafter, any kind of muscular activity that involves the legs, particularly the front thigh muscles, generates more dysmorphism. The skin over the front thighs becomes hugely infiltrated with cellulite tissue. All the key features are there—fluid retention, poor microcirculation and the formation of thick fibres. The more activity that is performed, the more this process continues and the larger the thighs become, particularly if the legs are exercised to the exclusion of other parts of the body. The increase in cellulite tissue associated with exercise of the front thigh muscles is the distinguishing factor in dysmorphism.

Dysmorphism is frequently seen in people who exercise the legs exclusively, or at least far more often than other parts of the body. Football, hill walking, kickboxing, step aerobics may all generate their fair share of dysmorphism. The end result is a slim body and tiny waist with little fat on the upper torso but a huge infiltration of cellulite tissue on the front thighs.

The condition is more noticeable in men than women. Men often notice the increase in the size of their thighs but rarely seek help. Try telling a man he has cellulite! In women, the condition is frequently confused with ordinary cellulite, although women with dysmorphism very often tend also to have cellulite elsewhere on the body. However, it's important to make the distinction between the two, since dysmorphism requires different treatment.

If sufferers continue to exercise without proper treatment, the problem will get progressively worse. On the other hand, simply ceasing to exercise is not the solution. Sure enough, the thighs will decrease in size, but the underlying problem will still be there. What is needed is a well-tailored exercise regime, combined with treatment to correct the microcirculatory and tissue-draining disorders.

- Digestive problems and stress can cause cellulite on the tummy in both men and women.
- Constant stress over a period of time can pull the bones of the neck and shoulders out of alignment and result in a fatty, cellulite-ridden lump on the nape of the neck, known as "Dowager's hump."
- Cellulite on the upper arms can arise from a disturbance in the venous drainage system and is almost always accompanied by cellulite elsewhere on the body.
- Dysmorphism, or footballer's legs, is a cellulite condition affecting the front thighs and can occur in both men and women, usually those who exercise the legs more frequently than the rest of the body.

5

So What Causes Cellulite?

Cellulite is primarily a lifestyle problem and may also be inherited

Now we know how cellulite is formed, but what are the factors that actually cause it? Well, these are varied, and this chapter outlines all the underlying causes. However, it is important to remember that, although cellulite begins with one or maybe two precipitating factors, it soon snowballs into one final common course. So, what may start as a fat storage or water retention problem can ultimately cause disruption to the microcirculation and the lymphatic and venous drainage. Think of it as an avalanche that starts off as a tiny snowfall which, when it gains sufficient momentum, eventually causes the whole mountainside to collapse, regardless of where the first flake fell. To get rid of the "avalanche" every bit of fallen snow has to be removed and, likewise, when treating cellulite we have to remove all the precipitating as well as the existing factors.

EXCESS CALORIES AND FAT STORAGE

Although cellulite does not discriminate between fat or thin people, fatter people do seem to be at greater risk since, after all, cellulite develops in fatty tissue. It makes sense, therefore, to take a good look at our diet and take steps to rectify any problems that may cause us to gain excess weight.

FAT

The body needs fat, but only in small quantities

Fat is essential for the normal functioning of the body. Hormones, cell membranes and nerves are made from fat and a certain amount of fat is necessary for warmth and protection. However, the amount of fat we actually need is quite small and excess fat from the diet is stored by the body in case of a future shortfall. The problem is that in the western world today, that shortfall never comes.

Yo-yo dieting and fat storage

In women, excess fat in the diet is preferentially taken up by the fat cells in the hips, thighs, bottom and knees. The relative surfeit of fat-storing receptors on the surface of these cells means that they are more ready to absorb fat, yet less likely to release it than fat cells on the upper body. Thus, any weight gained appears on the lower body and any weight lost comes off the upper body. Repeat dieting—the yo-yo syndrome—only worsens this scenario.

Diets with sugary or fatty "treats"

Furthermore, certain weight-reducing diets that allow "treats" of chocolate, cheese, biscuits—or whatever fatty or sugary confectionery you can lay your hands on—only compound this problem. Think about it. If you eat less, you will lose fat—eventually. So far, so good. But if you cheat or have a "treat," then what do you eat? Sugar or fat. Chocolate, cream, cakes, biscuits. All this does is satisfy your desire for these items, reward you for your efforts at dieting all day long, and then deposit fat in the very areas where you wish to get rid of it! Nonsense, isn't it?

Skipping meals and snacking

Skipping meals and then compensating by eating high-calorie snacks such as crisps, chocolate and biscuits allows exactly the same process to continue. Far better then to stick to a sensible diet plan, one that satisfies your hunger with good nutritious food so that you don't feel the need to cheat.

- Excess fat and sugar in the diet is stored as fat, mainly around the thighs and bottom.
- Yo-yo dieting removes fat from the upper body and deposits it on the lower body.

- Weight-loss diets with sugary or fatty treats exacerbate the pear-shaped distribution of fat.
- Skipping meals and substituting sugary and fatty snacks allows fat to be deposited on the lower body.

SUGAR

Excess sugar in the diet will ultimately be stored as fat

Excess sugar in the diet follows much the same pattern. Sugar is stored in the liver as glycogen as a short-term energy supply that the body can use easily and rapidly. When this store is full, excess sugar will be stored as fat, again preferentially in the fat cells on the lower body. Storage of fat is a relatively simple process in terms of cell function, but its removal from fat cells is far more difficult.

Sugar level control and trace elements

Sugar in the blood needs to be kept at a stable level. Too little sugar and the brain suffers from lack of its essential food source; too much and the sugar is toxic to the cells. It is the job of insulin, a hormone produced by the pancreas, to maintain a normal and stable blood sugar level, and it is insulin that controls the storage of excess sugar as fat. Insulin does not work alone but requires the help of minute amounts of the trace elements chromium, zinc, nickel and cobalt, otherwise known as oligoelements.

High-sugar diets, hypoglycaemia and fat storage

A diet rich in sugar can overload the sensitive sugar-control mechanism and reduce the level of these essential trace elements in the blood. This means the insulin has to work much harder and is therefore secreted in greater quantities in order to reduce the sugar level to normal.

As a result, the sugar-control mechanism becomes more clumsy and more heavy-handed which leads to fluctuations in the blood sugar level. What happens is that any sugar intake, such as eating a biscuit, leads to a rapid absorption of the sugar and a rise in the blood sugar level. The insulin overcompensates to reduce the level to normal, stores the excess sugar as fat and, subsequently, the blood sugar level falls again. The symptoms of low blood sugar are feeling unwell, faint, light-headed, moody and generally weak. In order to overcome these symptoms, the individual, quite understandably, eats more sugar, whereupon the vicious circle is continued. More sugar, more hunger. More hunger, more sugar—and more fat storage.

This condition is known as hypoglycaemia and occurs mainly as a result of a high sugar intake over a long period of time, but it is also often associated with a diet poor in trace elements.

A diet poor in trace elements

A diet that is rich in over-processed, ready-made and pre-packed foods and low in fresh fruit, vegetables, meat, nuts, pulses and fish can quickly lead to a deficiency in essential trace elements (oligoelements). A trace element deficiency is not always easy to diagnose, and the sufferer may not even be aware of the symptoms, as they arise very slowly and are commonly associated with fatigue, lack of energy and other rather vague symptoms. Such symptoms can easily be overlooked both by the individual and their doctor, and it is not until hypoglycaemia and sugar craving develop that a diagnosis is made.

Pre-menstrual sugar craving

Hypoglycaemia may also occur during the pre-menstrual period and be responsible for pre-menstrual sugar craving. While some research does suggest that women need an extra five hundred calories per day in the week before their period which could account for the sugar craving, other research indicates that the hormonal changes that occur pre-menstrually merely highlight the lack of B vitamins, magnesium, chromium and zinc. It may well be that both these hypotheses are true, depending on the individual's basic body nature and hormone sensitivity.

Moreover, very often the presence of one substance in the body can block or stimulate the absorption of another, and sugar eaten together with fat seems to stimulate the absorption of fat. Therefore eating foods such as chocolate, cakes, pastries and ice cream, which contain both fat and sugar, means that the fat is more readily absorbed than when fat and sugar are eaten separately.

- Excess sugar in the diet is stored initially as glycogen in the liver and then ultimately as fat on the lower body.
- Excess sugar in the diet can disturb the sugar control mechanism and lead to sugar craving and weight gain.
- A diet low in fresh, non-processed foods can lead to a defi-

ciency in the sugar-controlling trace elements chromium, zinc, nickel and cobalt.

- Pre-menstrual sugar craving may be due to a genuine need for extra calories.
- Pre-menstrual sugar craving may also be caused by hormonal changes which highlight a vitamin, mineral and trace element deficiency.

ALCOHOL

Alcohol is rich in calories but can be beneficial in small doses

Alcohol is an excellent stimulant of the microcirculation and therefore, theoretically, beneficial in small doses. Red wine, in particular, contains tannins derived from the grape skins which protect the microcirculation against damage from free radicals. However, alcohol is a rich source of calories which are rapidly stored as fat and rarely used as an energy source. One gram of fat provides nine calories and one gram of alcohol provides seven calories. On the other hand carbohydrate (for example, starch, sugar) and protein contain only four calories per gram, so we can see that alcohol is more akin to fat in the calorie stakes. It also weakens your resolve to stick to a sensible diet! In the cellulite war, alcohol has to be treated with respect.

- Alcohol is rich in calories and is rapidly turned into fat.
- Alcohol weakens your resolve to follow a diet.

WATER RETENTION

An excess intake of water is, contrary to popular belief, not a cure for cellulite. What is necessary is a balanced intake of sodium, protein, potassium and water.

Water is an essential nutrient for good health, and several bodily functions are dependent on it. The distribution of water in the body is regulated by the level of protein and the balance between sodium and potassium. Protein acts like a sponge to absorb the fluid and maintain an adequate level of water in the blood and circulation system. Sodium is also necessary for maintaining water in the blood and between the cells of the tissues, while potassium is responsible for maintaining the water levels within the cells themselves. A good intake of protein and a balanced intake of sodium and potassium is therefore necessary to maintain a healthy equilibrium.

SODIUM AND POTASSIUM

Sodium is found in salt and foods containing salt such as smoked, tinned, preserved and pre-packed foods as well as processed cheeses, meats and fish. We also tend to add salt liberally to fresh foods, either during cooking or at the table. Potassium, on the other hand, is found in fruit and vegetables, and many of us eat far too little of these foods. See how easy it is, therefore, to upset the sodium-potassium balance!

Too much salt in our diet can cause fluid retention in the blood and tissues. Normally, the body recognises that it has too much sodium on board and removes it through the kidneys. Sodium can also be lost through the skin as perspiration, which is why in hot weather we need to eat more salt to compensate. However, some people seem to have an inherited deficiency in removing excess sodium and tend to become overloaded with fluid. Gravity causes the fluid to settle in the legs, causing or making existing cellulite worse. Such people need to keep a careful watch on their intake of salt and salty foods, and ensure they eat plenty of fresh fruit and vegetables to obtain sufficient potassium to rectify the balance.

Even if you do not have an inherited deficiency, and there is no clinical way of detecting this at present, enormous amounts of sodium in the diet will still finally overload the kidneys and cause water retention. Water builds up in the tissues of the body, in particular the legs, again due to the effect of gravity.

WATER

An adequate water intake allows sufficient water to be equally distributed between the cells and tissue fluid. The amount of water in the body is regulated by the kidneys, which are able to detect the amount of sodium and water in the blood. Too much water and the kidneys make more urine, too little and you become thirsty and drink more.

However, the kidneys can only respond to what they are told—in other words, the level of water and sodium in the blood that reaches them. So, if in conditions of poor venous and lymphatic drainage, fluid leaks out of the blood into the surrounding tissues, the kidneys are unaware of this. The blood is still circulating and reaching the kidneys, albeit in a more concentrated form. Consequently, water trapped amongst the tissues remains undetected by the kidneys. Drinking more and more water merely adds to this process. The veins are leaky, the return of fluid to the heart is inadequate, and water collects in the tissues of the legs.

Furthermore, too little sodium or protein in the diet can just make this problem worse by not allowing sufficient water to be retained in the bloodstream.

DIURETICS

Diuretics, often prescribed for water retention, simply make the problem worse. Although diuretics will help in the treatment of water retention caused by a weak heart, they won't help water retention that results from an impaired lymphatic or venous drainage system. Some of the more commonly used diuretics allow potassium to leak out of the kidneys, thus further upsetting the body's sodium-potassium balance and ultimately causing more water retention. Such diuretics need to be supplemented by potassium in tablet form to re-establish the sodium-potassium balance, although this will not cure fluid retention and cellulite in the legs. In Part Two we will discuss better ways of stimulating the function of the veins and lymph vessels to improve the removal of fluid from the legs.

Some slimming pills also contain small amounts of diuretics which can also deplete the body of potassium. Lack of potassium only shows itself when the body is severely depleted. Fatigue and irritability are the main signs. The subtle effects of water retention are in force well before the clinical signs of low potassium are evident.

PROTEIN

Protein is found in meat, fish, eggs, milk, pulses, soya, nuts and cheese. Remember that nuts and some cheeses contain far too much fat to be of value in a cellulite control diet. Too little protein in our diet means that water is no longer held by the sponge-like action of protein in the blood and instead leaks out into the tissues. A diet rich in junk foods, fatty and/or sugary snacks and sweets, but with little protein, can easily contribute to low levels of protein in the body.

- Water distribution throughout the body depends on the balance of sodium and potassium and the level of protein.
- Some people are very sensitive to sodium in the diet and need to monitor their intake.
- Anyone who has an excess intake of sodium will ultimately suffer from water retention.

- Fresh fruit and vegetables are essential to maintain an adequate intake of potassium.
- Diuretics taken to cure water retention that is not associated with heart disease can deplete the body's stores of potassium.
- Diuretics do not help in the long term and frequently exacerbate the problem.

ARTIFICIAL FOOD PRODUCTS: COLOURINGS, FLAVOURINGS, PRESERVATIVES, PESTICIDES

Weight gain, fluid retention, tissue damage and circulatory disturbance may be caused by a high intake of artificial food products

The body has a system of enzymes that digest food and detoxify the toxins we consume in our daily diet, and these enzymes are "helped" by so-called antioxidant vitamins and minerals. This system has evolved over hundreds of years, hand in hand with the way our diet has developed. However, in recent years we have added literally thousands of new products to our diet in the form of colourings, flavourings, preservatives and the like. Unfortunately, we have added them at a rate that has outstripped the body's ability to develop enzymes to digest and detoxify them. Luckily, the body already has a number of enzymes that will adapt and do the job and, for the most part, our bodies manage very well. However, there are some situations where this adaptation system may not work.

The end result will be tissue damage and fluid retention caused by blocking the action of the detoxifying enzyme system and a build-up of artificial food products in the body. Fat storage and water retention causes weight gain, and this excess weight is often difficult to shift. The legs become swollen with retained fluid, and the veins, lymph vessels and microcirculation all become weakened by the effects of toxins and other unwanted products.

SENSITIVITY AND SUSCEPTIBILITY TO ARTIFICIAL FOOD PRODUCTS

Certain individuals are unable to detoxify artificial food products

In the first instance, it is estimated that about 20 per cent of people have a deficiency in certain detoxifying enzymes, which means they are unable to metabolise or detoxify certain artificial food products. Some of these people are already aware of their sensitivity to certain products because they suffer food or chemical allergies or other adverse effects and simply avoid the foods or chemicals which upset them. Monosodium glutamate, included in many processed foods and in Chinese food, is a common cause of upset. Not only are many people unable to metabolise it, it also has a high sodium content.

Secondly, it may be that the enzymes are present in normal amounts, but because the individual is eating so many artificial food products, their detoxifying system, however good, is simply overloaded.

Thirdly, some people are deficient in the antioxidant vitamins and minerals selenium, beta-carotene, vitamin C and vitamin E which means that the detoxifying enzymes are unable to work at their full capacity. A diet rich in processed foods and low in fresh fruit, vegetables, meat, fish and pulses will be lacking in these valuable antioxidants.

Finally, we do not know the full effects on the body of all the artificial products we are eating, particularly in the case of pre-packed, ready-made meals. Throughout the food processing chain, chemicals such as preservatives, colourings and flavourings are added. Because these are included in the ingredients listed on the packaging, it is relatively simple for us to avoid them if we choose to. However, other chemicals used in the storage, packaging and presentation of food may actually leak into the food itself. The big problem is that these chemicals are not listed along with the ingredients but, sure enough, they arrive in our food. These chemicals, too, require detoxification and may therefore overload an already overworked enzyme system.

We are only just beginning to appreciate the effect of all such chemicals on the body but there are still many unanswered questions. Much research is being done and it may be that these chemicals will turn out to be quite benign, but the truth is that, at present, we just don't know. Until we have the answers, it would be wise to avoid them.

- Artificial food products are not always properly metabolised by the body and may contribute to weight gain, fluid retention and cellulite.

ARTIFICIAL SWEETENERS

Artificial sweeteners contain no calories but may still cause weight gain

Artificial sweeteners such as aspartame, acesulfame K, saccharin and sorbitol also need to be detoxified by the body's enzyme system. However, they play an additional and interesting role in the development of fatty tissue and cellulite.

Again, it's a question of sensitivity. When we eat sugar, the taste buds on the tongue detect the sweetness and, in preparation for the increase in the blood sugar level, send a message to the pancreas to release insulin. Insulin, as we know, is the hormone responsible for maintaining a stable blood sugar level and also stimulates the storage of excess sugar as fat.

So, eating "normal" sugar produces a normal response; sugar enters the bloodstream and is dealt with by insulin. But because it is the initial sweet taste that triggers the release of insulin, in sensitive individuals artificial sweeteners can also induce the same response. However, since artificial sweeteners contain no calories, they cannot be stored as fat. The insulin is therefore unable to complete its task and "hangs around" in the system where it can interact with other hormones and cause water retention.

Even the mere act of looking at a delicious sugary food can trigger the secretion of insulin and hence water retention. So there may, after all, be some truth in the claim that some people only have to look at a cream cake to gain weight! However, this doesn't mean you have to cross the road to avoid the cake shop. You need to re-establish a normal sugar-insulin intake. More about this in Chapter 8.

- Artificial sweeteners in sensitive individuals cause weight gain by fluid retention.

FOOD ALLERGIES AND INTOLERANCE

Food allergies can lead to cellulite and therefore must be treated

Food allergies can cause "heavy" legs and water retention and lead to the development of cellulite. A small but significant number of women with cellulite suffer from food allergies and, conversely, many women with food allergies go on to develop cellulite. Therefore, it is important that such allergies are identified and treated if we are to successfully prevent or get rid of our cellulite.

There are various misconceptions that certain foods such as milk and milk products cause cellulite. Well, per se, they don't. But it is interesting that a milk-free diet does help many people to overcome cellulite. However, it's not the milk or milk product itself, but rather an allergy to milk that is to blame. Other common foods such as wheat, eggs, coffee and even tomatoes can all evoke the same reaction.

In recent years we have become more aware that the food we eat can cause health-related problems. Vague complaints such as tiredness, headaches, irritability, mood swings, abdominal pain, bloating, weight gain and water retention may all stem from allergies to certain foods. Food allergy or intolerance is a complex subject and full of apparent contradictions. How, for example, can you become allergic to a food that you eat every day and, very often, crave for? And how is it that certain symptoms seem to be relieved when the very same food is eaten?

A "true" food allergy in the strictest sense of the word involves the sudden and violent release of allergic substances in the body, causing a fairly rapid onset of symptoms that can be very unpleasant. Symptoms such as swelling of the mouth and skin, hives, nausea, vomiting and, in severe cases, anaphylactic shock (severe allergic reaction with collapse) appear almost immediately after eating the culprit food. The sufferer is thus able to easily identify the problem food and avoid it in the future. Of course, if they were to inadvertently eat that particular food again, then the symptoms would reappear with tell-tale reliability. Even a small quantity of the offending food could cause an allergic reaction.

Nowadays, we are more aware that other manifestations of allergic reactions to food may occur, but with less violent symptoms and less directly related to the culprit food. Although these are less easy to detect in a clinical setting or by blood or skin tests, they are nevertheless still food allergies. Some people prefer to call them food intolerances to differentiate between "true" food allergies and other food allergies.

Food intolerance, as we shall call it, can involve a wide range of seemingly unrelated symptoms, which is why it tends to evade diagnosis by even the most meticulous of doctors. In the long term, food intolerance can have far-reaching effects on the circulation system and the metabolism, which are central to the development of cellulite. About 20 per cent of my cellulite clients are intolerant to certain foods and respond well to a suitable diet, along with other treatment for the cellulite.

The most common symptoms are headache, migraine, fatigue, irritability, abdominal bloating, food cravings, weight gain or difficulty in losing weight, heavy legs and water retention. The symptoms tend to come and go, often according to the level of stress, tiredness or anxiety that a person is under rather than the amount of food eaten.

It is quite common for certain culprit foods to feature regularly in the diet without the sufferer being aware that they are intolerant to those particular foods. Wheat could be eaten at all three meals—cereal for breakfast, sandwich for lunch and pasta for the evening meal. Milk likewise—cereal with milk for breakfast, yoghurt at lunchtime, cheese at night and milk in tea or coffee during the day.

In other words, the diet alone may or may not give any clue. It is necessary to look at the combination of symptoms together with the diet and other factors such as past medical history, possible inheritance of an allergic disposition, the time-scale of the symptoms and if they are precipitated after eating or fasting. Biscuits, cheese, milk and chocolate as pick-me-ups may indicate an underlying food intolerance.

Very often, eating the offending food may appear to make the symptoms disappear, at least for a while. Indeed, the sufferer may even become "addicted" to the culprit food. In many ways, food intolerance and addiction is just like tobacco addiction; the culprit food, albeit harmful to us, is necessary to satisfy our craving. If we exclude that particular food from our diet, we suffer withdrawal symptoms and often crave the food in question to remove the unpleasant sensations. However, when we finally stop eating the problem food, after an initial withdrawal period, we feel better. Not just better, but much better. The symptoms that we have tolerated for ages get worse during the withdrawal period and then seem to melt away. Food withdrawal symptoms and ultimate improvement are significant pointers that food intolerance was the cause of the problem.

Adjusting your diet to treat a food intolerance may help prevent cellulite and also help get rid of existing cellulite more quickly. The treatment of cellulite due to food intolerance has to be thorough, scientifically based and tailored to each individual.

SYMPTOMS THAT CAN BE ASSOCIATED WITH FOOD INTOLERANCE

Digestive system: mouth ulcers, sore tongue, sore throat, indigestion, nausea, vomiting, abdominal pain, bloating, diarrhoea, constipation, colitis, irritable bowel syndrome

Head and nerves: headache, irritability, fatigue, depression, hyperactivity

Hormonal (cellulite-related): water retention, cellulite, weight gain, difficulty in losing weight, food cravings, weight swings

Joints and muscles: aching joints, arthritis, muscle fatigue, muscle pain

Respiratory system: sneezing, wheezing, asthma, coughing, post-nasal drip, runny nose, blocked nose, itchy nose, itchy eyes

Skin: eczema, urticaria (hives), itching, rashes

MOST COMMON CULPRIT FOODS

The most common foods that cause food intolerance are listed below. More practical advice is given in Chapter 8.

Alcohol	Milk
Apples	Oranges
Chicken	Potatoes
Chocolate	Tea
Coffee	Tomatoes
Corn	Wheat
Eggs	

POSSIBLE CAUSES OF FOOD INTOLERANCE

Food intolerance, like most medical conditions, tends to favour certain people. Such people often have a predisposition to develop food intolerance, and genetic make-up and inheritance play a large role. Below is a short list of predisposing factors that you can use as a checklist for self-diagnosis.

- Inheritance—one of your parents suffers from a classic allergic reaction such as hay fever, asthma, eczema, migraine or food allergy.
- Early introduction to bottle-feeding/ceasing breast-feeding.
- Poor diet—a diet with a high content of processed foods.
- Stress of any kind.
- Bowel infection, inflammation or damage.
- Certain viruses—in particular hepatitis A, glandular fever.

- Allergies and/or intolerance to certain foods in the diet can cause cellulite, weight gain and heavy legs.
- Intolerance to common foods shows itself as many symptoms, seemingly unrelated.
- You are more likely to be allergic to a food that you frequently eat such as wheat or milk.
- Treating the food allergy helps the treatment of cellulite.

HORMONAL INFLUENCES

Hormones, particularly relating to the female sex organs, can influence the development of cellulite

Fatty tissue in the lower body region can be affected by hormones such as oestrogen, progesterone and growth hormone. Cellulite, as we know, is predominantly a female problem and this is in part due to the role played by the female sex hormones, oestrogen and progesterone. Cellulite can develop in women from the early teens and continue to do so right up until the menopause is safely over. Although men can suffer from the condition known as dysmorphism (footballer's legs), they are not afflicted by "true" cellulite and this is due to the absence of female hormones.

OESTROGEN AND OTHER HORMONES

Oestrogen and progesterone can lead to cellulite

Oestrogen plays a part in the distribution of fat cells around the body and, in particular, controls the number of fat-storing and fat-releasing receptors on the cell surface during cell development. It encourages the development of fat-storing cells at puberty and stimulates their growth around the breasts, thighs, bottom and knees, which gives us the rounded features associated with femininity. Thus in periods of growth, oestrogen together with growth hormone will tend to encourage the laying down of fat cells in these areas. The muscles, bones, heart, lungs and fatty tissue also grow extremely quickly. This rapid growth often outstrips the ability of the skin to keep up which leads to the development of stretch marks. These are usually only seen in women and, of course, their appearance is most marked after periods of rapid growth such as puberty and pregnancy.

Large stretch marks suggest a huge burst of growth and are often the only pointer to be found when looking for a cause of cellulite. Rapid growth is often overlooked as a cause of cellulite in young women. Stretch marks on the legs, thighs and calves suggest a particularly rapid growth and fat deposition on the legs.

Exactly how oestrogen affects the fat cells is not fully understood, but we do know that it is a question of fatty tissue sensitivity to oestrogen rather than the level of oestrogen in the blood. There is no doubt that some women are more sensitive than others to oestrogen; some women can take the combined (oestrogen and progesterone) contraceptive pill with no ill-effects at all, while other women who are taking the same dosage feel quite unwell, swollen or uncomfortable. They may suffer migraines, headaches, depression as well as heavy legs and weight gain. In such cases, the fatty tissue responds to the hormones by storing fat, and the veins respond by slowing down their function, which may lead to the development of cellulite.

Likewise, progesterone, for example as in the progesterone-only or combined pill, may also play a part in the development of cellulite as progesterone can cause fluid retention, weight gain and weak veins, again only in progesterone-sensitive women.

The secretion of oestrogen and progesterone is controlled by two hormones known as luteinising hormone (LH) and follicle-stimulating hormone (FSH). According to research carried out in France, any alteration to the normal functioning of the ovaries can encourage the formation of cellulite. At present, this can be explained by a change in the relative levels of oestrogen, progesterone, LH and FSH or, more likely, a change in tissue sensitivity to these hormones.

During the normal menstrual cycle, LH and FSH are secreted by the pituitary gland situated in the brain. The ovaries respond by secreting oestrogen and progesterone which stimulate the lining of the womb. In turn, oestrogen released by the ovaries has a feedback effect on the pituitary gland so that the whole system regulates itself like a thermostat. This system is known as the ovarian-pituitary axis and represents the intimate relationship between the ovaries and the pituitary gland in the brain.

Unlike a thermostat, however, which turns off when the temperature reaches the required level, during the menstrual cycle the ovaries—and possibly other tissues as well—undergo a change in sensitivity so that the effects of LH and FSH may differ at certain times of the month. Sometimes the effects may be very strong, at other times they will be minimal. This is a complicated phenomenon, but it does help explain why minor changes to the ovaries can sometimes cause extreme oestrogen and progesterone sensitivity and why, at other times, they seem to have no effect.

Use of the contraceptive pill, infection, damage or inflammation of the internal gynaecological organs (salpingitis, sterilisation, pelvic inflammatory disease, for example) may all contribute to altering the working of the delicate thermostat.

This scenario of events is at best an educated guess since, although it is fairly easy to measure hormone levels, it is not easy to measure tissue sensitivity to varying hormone levels. There are, however, certain clinical conditions that lend weight to these theories. In very young women (early to mid-teens), the introduction of the contraceptive pill can interfere with the LH-FSH influence on the immature ovaries and is more likely to cause cellulite than in the case of an older woman (twenties onwards) who has a more mature, and thus more stable, ovarian-pituitary axis. Similarly, at the opposite end of the reproductive system, the introduction of hormone replacement therapy (HRT) to a menopausal, and thus equally fragile, ovarian-pituitary axis, can also cause very stubborn cellulite.

Therefore, any interference to the ovarian-pituitary axis at times when it is immature, fragile or menopausal as a result of the contraceptive pill, HRT, or gynaecological surgery, infection or inflammation, will cause cellulite, and such cellulite is particularly resistant to treatment.

Treatment for infertility, which involves the use of ovary-stimulating drugs, may also cause the development of stubborn cellulite. Again, this is due to an interference in the ovarian-pituitary axis by high-dose ovarian stimulants, causing increased tissue sensitivity to oestrogen and, thus, increased fat storage.

- Oestrogen and progesterone are female hormones. Both may be used in the combined contraceptive pill. Progesterone also appears in the progesterone-only pill.
- Oestrogen stimulates fat storage in the breasts, thighs, bottom, hips and knees; this effect is seen most at puberty and during pregnancy.
- Progesterone (for example, in the mini pill and combined pill) may cause fluid retention.
- Infection, inflammation and any disturbance in the ovaries and gynaecological organs can lead to cellulite.
- HRT can cause cellulite and also render existing cellulite difficult to treat.

PELVIC SURGERY

Surgery to the pelvic area is often a cause of cellulite and weight gain

Pelvic surgery, particularly to the gynaecological system, can disrupt the lymphatic return. There is no doubt that many women experience a weight gain after undergoing a hysterectomy and some women also after sterilisation. Many doctors claim that this is due to a release from the constant fear of pregnancy. Damage to the abdominal muscles is also cited as a reason for the weight gain and loss of shape after such operations, although lost muscle can be regained through exercise.

However, these explanations are not enough to account for the weight gain on the lower legs. The most important reason—and the most overlooked—is a disruption to the lymphatic drainage system due to interference with the anatomy of the pelvis, either during the actual surgery or the events that follow. Fibrous tissue is laid down as a reaction to the cutting, burning and bleeding that occurs during surgery. This tissue is tough and inelastic, like gristle, and has no regard for existing boundaries or structures. Sometimes the fibrous tissue forms restrictive bands around the delicate lymphatic vessels, causing damage and fluid retention in the legs. These thick, restrictive bands are known as adhesions and when they cause severe problems have to be surgically removed.

Pelvic surgery, like any other operation, is another stress and may also interfere with the ovarian-pituitary axis.

- Pelvic surgery may disrupt the lymphatic return and cause cellulite.

PREGNANCY

Pregnancy can cause fluid retention and fat storage and may lead to cellulite

Pregnancy has a profound effect on several bodily systems and is often, but not always, a cause of cellulite.

During the months preceding the birth, the womb increases in size and presses upon the lymph vessels and veins. The result is a reduction in the drainage of lymph and blood from the tissues, thus setting the scene for fluid retention and the development of cellulite. This situation is temporary, and immediately after the birth, the pressure on the draining vessels is reduced and the flow is restored to normal.

However, during the time of limited drainage, fluid—particularly lymph fluid—has been accumulating in the tissues and beginning to form fibres. Oestrogen, progesterone and other hormones are secreted in huge amounts in order to support the developing foetus. These hormones affect the storage of fat and fluid—the fat tends to be stored around the legs, thighs and bottom in response to the rising oestrogen levels.

The developing foetus requires iodine for the formation of its own thyroid gland. The thyroid gland controls cell metabolism and the rate at which energy (fat) is burned off. The foetus takes as much iodine as it needs from the mother. Depending on her iodine stores and the status of her own thyroid, the mother may herself then suffer a deficiency of iodine. Consequently, her thyroid may not function 100 per cent and she will be unable to burn off the fat stored during pregnancy. Often this shows not in the first pregnancy but in subsequent pregnancies where each one adds a few extra pounds that are resistant to all efforts at removal. In this case, iodine supplements are necessary to restore the normal thyroid function and aid return to pre-pregnancy weight.

Pregnancy is not all bad news, however. Recent research has shown that breast-feeding is a very effective way, in fact the only way, of removing excess fat on the lower part of the body after pregnancy. This is due to the fat-removing effect of the hormones involved in breast-feeding.

- Pregnancy is a high-oestrogen and progesterone state and the effects of these hormones are therefore multiplied.
- Pregnancy can cause fluid retention which may set the scene for the development of cellulite.
- Pregnancy can reduce the mother's stores of iodine, compromise the thyroid function and prevent a return to pre-pregnancy weight.
- Breast-feeding stimulates the hormones that reduce fat on the lower body.

ADRENALINE AND STRESS

Prolonged stress can lead to cellulite on the upper tummy and back of the neck as well as on the lower body

Adrenaline, a hormone produced by the adrenal gland, is secreted under conditions of fear, panic, anxiety or stress. This provides us with a physiological boost to overcome the adverse force with which we are dealing; the heart rate increases, more oxygen is taken up by the lungs, the muscles receive more blood, and sugar is produced from stored fat so that we have the sudden energy and strength to overcome the situation or run like crazy away from it. This is quite a normal reaction and is known as the "flight or fight" syndrome.

However, prolonged stress over a continuous period of time can affect us in different ways. Some people become a bag of nerves, exhibiting all the outward signs of very active adrenal glands: rapid heartrate, staring eyes, over-breathing, trembling. Such people tend to be thin because of all the nervous energy they are burning up. In other people, the effect is quite the reverse. Instead of releasing sugar from the fat cells, the surge of adrenaline actually makes them store more fat, mostly on the thighs, bottom and hips.

Some people under conditions of stress also store fat in the common stress areas, on the upper part of the tummy, just beneath the ribs and above the tummy button, or on the back of the neck—known rather unattractively as "Dowager's hump." Furthermore, because of the stress involved, the neck is often the seat of arthritis, pain and spasm; such people frequently suffer chronic neck pain, arm pain, headaches and migraines. In these cases, it is necessary to treat the neck problem through osteopathy, therapeutic massage, chiropractic or mesotherapy (a local skin injection technique) in addition to any treatment for cellulite.

However longstanding the stress and however irresolvable it seems, it is essential that it is treated or at least its effects minimised by stress-reducing therapies (see Chapters 9 and 10).

• Adrenaline normally causes weight loss but can actually cause weight gain in some women.
• Stress is a major cause of cellulite and must be treated.

DIRECT DAMAGE TO THE LYMPHATIC SYSTEM, MICROCIRCULATION AND VENOUS RETURN

Any damage to the lymphatic system, microcirculation or venous return will inevitably lead to cellulite

As lymphatic drainage, microcirculation and venous return are closely interrelated once the vessels are deep in the tissues, it's simpler to consider them as a whole when looking at the causes of cellulite.

As we now know, a good circulation and lymphatic system is important for maintaining the health of fatty tissue. Once the lymph fluid from the blood has completed its task of supplying the cells with oxygen and nutrients, it needs to be drained away via the lymph vessels.

Since the walls of the lymph vessels have no muscles, they rely on three main mechanisms to pump fluid out of the tissues and back to the heart. These are the pumping action of the leg muscles, the contracting and expanding of the diaphragm (thoraco-abdominal pump) and the plantar return reflex which originates in the sole of the foot.

BLOCKAGE OF THE LYMPH NODES THROUGH CONSTIPATION, INFECTION OR INFLAMMATION

Chronic pelvic infections and constipation can lead to cellulite

The lymph vessels, like the veins, join up to form larger and larger vessels that eventually enter the blood circulation as the blood flows back to the heart. But before the lymph fluid returns to the blood, it passes through numerous small lymph nodes that act as a filter to cleanse the fluid of waste products and impurities. However, there are several factors that can impede the flow of lymph and almost all lead to cellulite.

Constipation and pelvic infection or inflammation can cause the lymph nodes to get larger as they prepare to filter and remove the infecting or obstructing agent from the lymph fluid. The flow of lymph slows down, creating a temporary backlog. This backlog is normally resolved quite quickly so that no long-term damage occurs. However, after a longstanding infection or inflammation of the pelvis, or continued constipation, irritable bowel syndrome, chronic bowel or gynaecological infection, the backlog can be transferred back to the tissues and cause fluid retention and cellulite.

There is a further consequence of constipation in terms of cellulite. Constipation fills the bowel with waste products that should have long been removed. There is a limit to the volume to which the bowel can expand to accommodate the additional contents, and the extra volume will cause the bowel to press on the lymph vessels in the pelvis and thus retard their normal function.

- Constipation and infection or inflammation of the legs or pelvis can cause the lymph nodes to enlarge and slow down the flow of lymph.
- Constipation can also cause cellulite as a result of pressure placed on the lymph vessels.

RESTRICTION OF THE NORMAL FLOW OF LYMPH; TIGHT CLOTHING

Lymph vessels can be compromised from both the outside and inside of the body

On their way back to the heart, the lymph vessels follow the same anatomical course as the arteries and veins. At the point where the arteries enter the legs to carry the blood supply, and the veins and lymph leave the legs to drain away the fluid, they pass through a very narrow channel in the groin, known as the inguinal canal.

The inguinal canal contains the femoral artery (the main artery in the thigh), the femoral vein, lymph vessels, nerves, fatty tissue and a few lymph nodes. Because the canal is so narrow and is covered in a tough coating of ligament, any outside pressure placed on this area, such as wearing tight jeans, can "squash" the channel, thus compromising its contents. The result is that the all-important lymph vessels and veins, with their weak walls, become squashed and are unable to drain fluid properly from the legs. The arterial wall, however, is tough and muscular and able to resist such pressure, and therefore the femoral artery manages perfectly well to continue supplying blood to the legs.

Tight jeans, hold-ups and tight underwear elastic will all contribute to the blockage or at least a slowing down of the return of lymph and venous blood from the legs. Sitting down while wearing tight clothing makes the problem worse and further slows down the flow.

• Tight clothing can place pressure on the inguinal canal and affect the venous and lymphatic drainage.

POOR POSTURE

Poor posture is a frequently overlooked cause of cellulite

The way we stand can affect the tightness of the inguinal canal. If we stand with a bad posture, pelvis tilted forwards (bottom sticking out, tummy forwards, abdominal muscles relaxed or sagging), this creates an exaggerated curve in the small of the back, known as lumbar lordosis, which compresses the contents of the inguinal canal, in particular the lymph vessels and veins. This results in an impaired venous and lymphatic return. Sagging abdominal muscles will not allow the thoraco-abdominal pump to function properly, if at all, which means that fluid will collect in the legs and the

bottom. Many Afro-Caribbean women suffer from lumbar lordosis, which is why many of them tend to have big bottoms and
thighs enormously infiltrated with cellulite. This cellulite, how-
ver, is quite treatable, providing the posture is improved.

Wearing high heels (over 2 inches high) will also cause the
pelvis to tip forwards or exaggerate the already prominent tilt.
Take care when choosing footwear.

Poor posture can squash the inguinal canal and disrupt lymphatic and venous return.
Sagging abdominal muscles can impede the function of the thoraco-abdominal pump and lead to fluid retention in the legs and
bottom.

ABDOMINAL BLOATING

Bloating is unsightly and unpleasant and can lead to cellulite

Abdominal bloating, wind and flatulence can indirectly influence
the development of cellulite. Bloating occurs when there is a retention of gas in the intestines which cause them to "blow up" like a
balloon. It is painful and unsightly, but there are remedies.

The "bloating" of the abdomen presses on the abdominal muscles, causing them to sag. The pelvis tips forwards and the tummy
sticks out, again placing pressure on the inguinal canal and dis-
rupting the return of lymph and venous blood to the heart. This situation can easily cause fluid retention in the legs and ultimately
lead to cellulite. In severe cases, wind in the intestines presses on
the diaphragm, preventing normal respiration and impairing the
function of the thoraco-abdominal pump, again leading to a build-
up of fluid in the bottom and thighs.

Constipation, poor digestion, food intolerance and abnormal gut
flora can contribute to abdominal bloating.

• Abdominal bloating can cause cellulite by compressing the
  inguinal canal and preventing the thoraco-abdominal pump
  from working properly.

MASSAGE

The wrong type of massage can damage the delicate lymph vessels

Massage performed incorrectly is extremely traumatic to the tissues. The delicate lymph vessels are easily damaged and excess pressure placed on them can cause them to go into spasm or even to rupture. In unhealthy tissue that is already congested and weakened by the cellulite process, the lymph vessels are even more fragile and more susceptible to damage. The lymph vessels can very easily go into spasm so that they fail to drain the lymph effectively. In some cases they can break, in which case their contents spill out into the very tissues they are trying to drain.

Massage to the tissues therefore should be very gentle, and it should not cause any reddening or discomfort and certainly no bruising. Only one type of massage is suitable to the treatment of cellulite, and this is a gentle technique known as Manual Lymph Drainage which respects the fragility and anatomy of the vessels. *All other forms of massage may simply be of no benefit and, at worst, harm the tissues.*

- Forceful massage techniques can place excessive pressure on the fragile lymph vessels and cause damage to the tissues.

INACTIVE OR SEDENTARY LIFESTYLE

Inactivity and too much sitting around can cause and prolong cellulite in several ways

An inactive or sedentary lifestyle can have repercussions on the lymphatic, microcirculatory and venous systems as well as causing weight gain—all of which can precipitate cellulite.

The lymph vessels rely on the pumping action of the leg muscles, the thoraco-abdominal pump and the plantar return reflex to stimulate the return of lymph to the blood, and an inactive body will simply not allow this return system to work. During our waking hours, over a period of a day, there will be a gradual increase in fluid held in the tissues of the legs. The increase in fluid stretches the skin and tissues—it's like stretching a woolly jumper—which then cannot regain their original elasticity. Overstretched, inelastic tissues allow further fluid retention. Protein-rich fluid in the tissues will eventually form fibrous tissue, and the accumulation of venous blood damages the capillary walls causing blood to leak into the tissues and cause further harm.

Sitting for prolonged periods of time puts pressure on the thighs and bottom, preventing blood flow to this area and damaging the fragile capillaries. The pressure on these small vessels prevents blood from properly irrigating the tissues with oxygen and nutrients, while the damage to the capillaries causes blood and lymph to leak into the tissues.

Damage to the microcirculation, inflammation of capillary walls and leakage of blood and lymph into the tissues is the first step in the development of cellulite. Such microscopic change caused by sitting will of course repair itself over time and, as a single factor, it may not cause any long-term damage. But remember that, although a sedentary lifestyle in itself may not be the precipitating factor, it can play a large part when other factors are also present and the "avalanche" of cellulite starts to build up.

- A sedentary lifestyle can have far-reaching consequences on the lymphatic, microcirculatory and venous systems and lead to the development of cellulite.

AIR TRAVEL

Inactivity and a change in atmospheric pressure can damage the lymphatic and circulatory systems

Any prolonged period of inactivity combined with a change in atmospheric pressure can allow fluid to leak more easily into the surrounding tissue, which is particularly damaging to the lymphatic and circulatory systems. Sitting down for a long period of time allows fluid to collect in the legs and is most frequently experienced as puffy, swollen or painful ankles after a long flight.

- Prolonged inactivity combined with a decompression in atmosphere allows fluid to leak from the circulation and into the tissues.

FREE RADICALS

Free radicals are extremely damaging to the body and may also contribute to the development of cellulite

Free radicals are highly charged molecules of oxygen that react very quickly and violently with cell components, thus damaging them. Free radicals are produced by the action of the sun, irradiation, chemicals in our food, but the most common source is smoking. Because of their intensely harmful effects, they play an important part in the ageing process, causing sun damage, cancer and degenerative diseases. Free radicals also cause damage to the walls of the small vessels resulting in inflammation and a leakage of blood and lymph fluid into the surrounding tissues.

• Free radicals from pollution, sunlight and smoking cause damage to the microcirculation.

SMOKING

Smoking is one of the most common sources of free radicals

Yes, smoking again! This is important, so it merits an entry of its own. Smoking is a double-edged sword since it causes damage to the microcirculation and also to the larger vessels as a result both of the free radicals generated and the chemical effect of the nicotine. Nicotine is a vasoconstrictor, which means it causes the small blood vessels to constrict. The smaller the vessel, then the less the amount of blood that can flow through it. Furthermore, you cannot totally compensate for the adverse effects that smoking has on the blood vessels by taking increased exercise. You may feel fit, even though you do smoke, but the state of your microcirculation will only be slightly better than a smoker who does no exercise at all.

• Nicotine is a vasoconstrictor and damages the microcirculation.

CAFFEINE

Too much caffeine can restrict the blood supply to the tissues but a small amount can be beneficial

Caffeine is a stimulant that increases mental awareness and aids concentration. It also increases the basal metabolic rate (the rate at which we burn calories) by about five per cent, thus aiding the removal of fat if combined with a weight-loss diet. However, caffeine has undesirable effects on the microcirculation since, taken in high doses, it is a vasoconstrictor and diminishes the amount of blood that reaches the fatty tissues.

Caffeine has to be treated with respect—take just enough and the metabolic rate increases, but take too much and the blood supply is affected. In general, the equivalent of one expresso should provide sufficient caffeine to stimulate your mind without affecting the blood vessels to any great degree.

- Caffeine in small doses increases the basal metabolic rate but in higher doses it damages the microcirculation.

LIPOSUCTION AND LIPOSCULPTURE

Liposuction and liposculpture are useful techniques for removing fat but can cause or worsen existing cellulite if performed incorrectly

Liposuction and liposculpture were once thought to be cures for cellulite but, at last, people are beginning to realise that this is not the case. When performed correctly, these techniques are effective ways of reshaping the body. As we now know, fatty tissue is extremely resistant to our efforts at reducing from the lower body and is preferentially removed from the upper torso. Cosmetic surgery provides a "quick fix" solution to this problem and can give excellent results, but certain areas of the body fare better than others. Particularly good results are seen with the inner thighs and inner knees.

However, liposuction or liposculpture performed on the outer or back part of the thighs can damage the fine network of capillaries and lymph vessels and set the scene for the development of cellulite. Sure enough, the thighs will be beautiful, slim, lean—for a while—until the microcirculation begins to complain and cellulite sets in. Only surgery to the inner knees and inner thighs, correctly performed by a skilled surgeon, will give good, long-lasting results—providing you don't fall back into unhealthy eating or exercise habits.

- Liposuction and liposculpture can remove fat but not cure cellulite.
- Liposuction and liposculpture must be performed with skill and restraint or they can cause or make existing cellulite worse.

BASIC BODY SHAPE AND GENETIC MAKE-UP

Your basic body shape may influence the development of cellulite

Do certain body shapes have a tendency to develop cellulite more easily than others? Are slim people less likely to get cellulite than those who are overweight? Well, I'm afraid that, as in any of the life sciences, nothing is straightforward. There are so many confusing variables and, at best, we can only speculate.

It may be true that certain body shapes are less likely to suffer from cellulite; generally, slim women do seem to be less troubled than plumper women, but this is by no means a hard and fast rule. What seems more likely is that, regardless of how thin or fat you are, if certain conditions prevail within the body, then cellulite will develop. However, with some body shapes, cellulite may develop more slowly or clear up more quickly than in others. Certainly women who have a muscular, stocky build find cellulite removal more of a problem than leaner, taller women.

GENETICS

Cellulite may be an inherited condition

Thankfully, cellulite does not affect everyone. Some women, whatever their size, seem destined to develop orange-peel thighs, while others will keep their sleek thighs all their life. Young women with cellulite may recognise the same tell-tale signs on their mothers' legs. So we do know that, to some degree, heredity can come into play—if your mother suffers from cellulite, then there's a good chance you will suffer too.

It's not that you actually inherit cellulite itself but rather the *potential* to develop cellulite. Some people unfortunately simply inherit a higher proportion of fat-storing fat cells, weak veins, lymph vessels, poor circulation or a sensitivity to oestrogen and other female hormones. Take a look at your family history. The features to look for are overweight, varicose veins, haemorrhoids, swollen ankles, cold feet and broken veins. Although you may inherit one or more of these factors, it is only later that you enhance your potential to develop cellulite by adding more factors, more snowballs to your growing avalanche.

- Cellulite may form more slowly or clear up more quickly in tall, lean women than in women with a stocky, muscular build.
- Hereditary factors may play a role in the development of cellulite.

6

ASSESSING YOUR CELLULITE

Now you know how cellulite is formed and the underlying factors that may precipitate it. But before you can decide how best to treat it, first it's important to know how your cellulite fits into the overall pattern of your body harmony. It's not enough to simply know you have cellulite; you need to know everything you can about the problem in hand—how much of it is fat, how much is cellulite and if there is a degree of dysmorphism? Then you need to establish how it started, how it has progressed and how it has responded to various factors in your lifestyle. What are the risk factors, what factors aggravate it, what attempts— if any—have you made to treat it and what was the outcome? Have you done everything possible to help yourself? In other words, you need to know—and face—the facts!

Only when you know all there is to know about the nature and history of your specific complaint and associated factors can you start to plan a suitable treatment regime. This chapter takes the form of a series of questions and answers, and answering the questions will help you decide on the best course of action. Specific advice on treatment can be found in Part Two. There is no overnight cure, no magic solution—you just need patience, motivation and dedication.

IS IT REALLY CELLULITE?

What are the signs of cellulite and how do these differ from ordinary fat?

There are a few medical investigation techniques that can reveal the presence of cellulite. These are expensive, time-consuming and often produce no better results than the well-trained eye.

As about ninety-five per cent of women suffer from cellulite, it could be argued that cellulite is a normal phenomenon. Some women tolerate it, others despise it. It depends on the degree of infiltration and your own attitude towards it. However, because cellulite can ultimately be successfully treated, I personally do not think we should accept that it is a "normal" feature of the adult female.

SELF-DIAGNOSIS

Cellulite can be diagnosed by using the skin-pinch and roll technique. To do this, gently take a large fold of normal, non-cellulite skin and rub it between your thumb and forefinger. You will see that the skin and underlying subcutaneous tissue is quite smooth. Depending on how much fat you have, the subcutaneous tissue will be almost absent, thin, or slightly thicker. It is fat that determines the thickness of the tissue, and what you are feeling is normal fatty tissue.

Now repeat the above test on the areas of the body where you suspect cellulite, for instance, the bottom, thighs and knees. You may need a mirror to examine your bottom properly or, alternatively, ask a close friend to help! If cellulite is present you will be able to recognise the symptoms in one or more of the stages described below which correspond to those in Chapter 3. Remember, cellulite develops gradually and there are a number of stages in its progression. The following stages are cumulative and so, for instance, if you recognise symptoms in stage four, you will also exhibit all or most of the symptoms in stages one to three, and so on.

Stage one: skin slow to heal; other signs not detectable

This is the pre-cellulite stage where the scene is set for its development. This tissue will show no visible signs of cellulite, although bruises and cuts may be slow to heal.

Stage two: fluid retention; broken veins; discolouration; skin thicker and slightly tender; easy bruising

Close examination of the skin reveals the tiniest broken veins and skin discolouration. The discolouration is caused by the broken veins allowing blood to enter the tissues. Bruises may appear after the smallest of knocks. When pinched gently between the forefinger and thumb, the skin itself feels thicker and perhaps slightly tender and you will see signs of orange-peel skin.

Stage three: orange-peel skin

Without pinching the skin, you will see evidence of fluid retention on its surface. The retained fluid causes the skin surrounding the hair follicles and sweat glands to push outwards, creating that familiar orange-peel appearance on the skin.

Stage four: tethering; mattress skin; skin cold to the touch; larger veins broken; spontaneous bruising

The skin now appears tethered, puckered, with or without pinching, known as "mattress skin". To feel, the skin is cold. Broken veins may be present and, if so, these will be quite large and often clearly visible on the skin below the cellulite areas. Bruising occurs spontaneously as well as after trivial knocks.

Stage five: hot islands of tissue

When you touch the skin you can feel areas of hot—not just warm—tissue amongst areas of cold tissue.

Stage six: steatomes

Large areas of fat are encased and tethered by fibres, forming steatomes which distort the normal silhouette.

The verdict

If you did not recognise any of the above symptoms, you can relax—you don't have cellulite. If you recognised the earlier symptoms but not the later ones, this suggests that your cellulite is in the relatively early stages of development. This means the cellular disturbance will be less advanced and is therefore likely to respond more rapidly to anti-cellulite measures.

If you see evidence of the later symptoms (stages five and six), this suggests that the cellulite is further advanced and pretty well established, with the formation of steatomes and hot islands of malnourished and poorly drained tissue. Such cellulite will almost certainly need medical intervention in order to be completely shifted. In this instance, be realistic and seek outside help as soon as possible. Misguided attempts at self-treatment will only lead to constant failure and frustration so that you are unlikely to stick with any future regime. Yo-yo dieting and subsequent fluctuations in weight will only make the cellulite worse.

So, once you have established that you definitely do have some cellulite, you need to know more about its distribution around the body and other factors that are contributing to it.

WHERE IS IT?

The distribution of cellulite around the body may affect the type of treatment that is required

Cellulite tends to form most frequently around the bottom, thighs, knees, lower legs and ankles but also on the tummy, upper arms and neck. Certain areas respond better than others to treatment and some areas require different forms of treatment. It is important to know this before you start any course of treatment.

First, make a note of the areas that are affected:

- Back thighs
- Outer thighs
- Bottom
- Front thighs
- Knees
- Lower legs and ankles
- Tummy
- Upper arms
- Neck

BACK THIGHS, OUTER THIGHS AND BOTTOM

The backs of the thighs, the area running from just beneath the bottom to just above the depression at the back of the knee, is the most common site for cellulite. The good news is that, although cellulite may develop more rapidly here, it will also respond more rapidly to intervention.

The outer thighs—where some people develop so-called "horse thighs"—and the bottom are the next most frequent sites, and these too respond fairly well to basic treatment, often without the need for medical intervention.

FRONT THIGHS

The front part of the thighs, from the groin to the kneecap, is the area that is often affected by dysmorphism. The diagnosis of dysmorphism is supported by a noticeable difference between the size of the upper body and the thighs. When dysmorphism is present, the thighs will be much bigger in comparison, creating a disproportionate shape. A badly planned exercise routine will exacerbate rather than cure dysmorphism, and if you continue to exercise the legs but not the rest of the body, the thighs will simply become bigger rather than leaner. Treatment requires a well-balanced diet and exercise regime, plus attention to the microcirculation, veins and lymphatic drainage, such as by MLD or mesotherapy.

KNEES

Heavy knees are often, but not always, associated with hormonal treatments such as HRT, the contraceptive pill and infertility treatment. It's not always easy to change the shape of the knees, so patience here is a virtue. Heavy knees need to be treated with respect when exercising. Allowing them to wobble about uncontrollably damages the lymph vessels and makes the cellulite worse, so always wear well-supporting lycra leggings or tights when exercising.

Many women find a pocket of cellulite on the inner area of the knees. This cellulite is often stubborn and difficult to remove due to an increased concentration of fibres in the cellulite tissue. If the cellulite is really stubborn, liposuction and liposculpture can give very good results here in removing the fat, especially if the pocket of fat is quite distinct and noticeable. However, they will not cure cellulite.

LOWER LEGS AND ANKLES

Cellulite on the lower legs, ankles and shins is almost always accompanied by cellulite elsewhere on the legs. Again, treatment will require patience and dedication. Interestingly, treatment of cellulite on the upper legs in the form of applied medical and massage techniques almost always removes cellulite on the lower legs.

TUMMY

Although most women have a stubborn layer of fat on the lower tummy, cellulite can settle anywhere on the abdomen from between the ribcage and the pubic bone. Nerves that connect the digestive organs to the skin on the abdomen can "translate" disorders such as irritable bowel syndrome, constipation or bloating onto the skin in the form of pain, tenderness, swelling and fluid retention.

The next time you have any pain in your tummy, gently pinch the skin on your tummy between your thumb and index finger. You should feel patches of skin that are tender, and this is due to these nerve connections. Cellulite treatment must be accompanied by treatment for the intestinal or digestive disorder.

The area just below the ribcage is a common stress area, and quite troublesome cellulite can form here as a result of adrenaline released under conditions of stress. Therefore, for any anti-cellulite treatment to be effective, it must be used in conjunction with measures to reduce the stress.

There are many methods of dealing with stress, so select the one that best suits you. Choose from yoga, relaxation techniques, Manual Lymph Drainage, aromatherapy, dance, exercise and stress counselling.

Men tend to suffer more frequently than women with the problem of cellulite on the tummy. The treatment for men is simpler because they do not have to grapple with the female hormones that encourage the deposition of fat in women. Getting men to admit that they may have cellulite in the first place is perhaps the main hurdle!

UPPER ARMS

Cellulite may also develop on the upper arms, usually in conjunction with cellulite elsewhere. This almost always suggests a general dysfunction in the small blood vessels, particularly in the veins.

The arms generally respond better than the legs to treatment, because the lymphatic and venous drainage systems here do not have to contend with gravity. If you treat the cellulite on other areas of the body through diet, exercise and nutritional supplements, you should find that the arms will improve without the need for specific treatment.

However, if your arms are particularly large or the cellulite is quite troublesome, then you might consider localised treatment in the form of creams and aromatherapy. Choose ones containing ingredients that will improve the venous drainage system (see Chapter 10).

Certainly, with my patients, I prefer not to treat the arms. I find that if I treat any accompanying cellulite on the legs and/or tummy, using creams and mesotherapy mixtures specifically aimed at improving the veins, then the arms heal themselves. This suggests that such products are not only absorbed through the skin and into the underlying tissue but that they are also absorbed to some extent into the general circulation to improve the function of the arteries, veins and lymph vessels throughout the body.

NECK

Cellulite on the neck arises from an underlying problem with the bones of the neck and surrounding muscles, as a result of prolonged stress. It stands to reason therefore that the underlying neck problem needs to be treated along with measures to deal with the stress.

Osteopathy, chiropractic, therapeutic massage, acupuncture, mesotherapy, relaxation techniques, Alexander technique, Pilates and specific exercises will all help longstanding neck problems. Try one of these as your first line of treatment. There is no point trying to lose weight, taking nutritional supplements or even applying cream to the neck until you have first sorted out the bone and muscle dysfunction. They simply won't help to get rid of cellulite on the neck.

CELLULITE—YOUR AID TO DIAGNOSIS

Site of cellulite	Possible underlying problem
Legs and bottom	Poor venous function
	Poor lymphatic return
	Poor or damaged microcirculation
	Excess fat storage
Front thighs	Dysmorphism
	with or without:
	poor venous function
	poor lymphatic return

	poor or damaged microcirculation
	excess fat storage
Tummy	Digestive problem such as
	constipation, irritable bowel syndrome
	Stress
	with or without:
	poor venous function
	poor lymphatic return
	poor or damaged microcirculation
	excess fat storage
Arms	Poor venous function
	with or without:
	poor or damaged microcirculation
	poor lymphatic return
	excess fat storage
Neck	Bone or muscle problem such as arthritis, neck
	pain, muscle spasm
	Stress

HOW AND WHEN DID IT START?

It is important to establish when your cellulite started and to identify the factors that caused it

The longer you have had cellulite, the longer it has had to establish itself and the longer it will take to shift. If you have had cellulite for some time, you'll need to prepare yourself for a lengthy battle, but don't give up. Be patient and don't expect it to disappear overnight. Motivation is the key.

It is important to establish when your cellulite first started and what the precipitating factors were if you are to effectively deal with it.

PRECIPITATING FACTORS

Poor diet	Junk foods, high-calorie foods, chocolate, etc.
Inactivity or decrease in activity	Starting college or a sedentary job

Hormonal influences:

At puberty	No contraceptive pill usage
	Contraceptive pill usage
After pregnancy	First pregnancy
	Subsequent pregnancy
Hormone replacement	Therapy
Stress	Change of home, emotional or work circumstances
No particular event but family history	Family history of cellulite, heavy legs, bad circulation, fluid retention.

If you can pinpoint a specific event that caused your cellulite, then so much the better. By identifying the initial cause, at least you can take steps to treat it. And, as long as you remove the precipitating factor, the more likely you will rid yourself of cellulite for good. Without doubt, cellulite is more difficult to treat if the original cause, whether it be stress, anxiety or a poor diet, is not dealt with. Remember, once cellulite has set in, you have to treat *all* known causes.

If cellulite developed at puberty in the absence of other precipitating factors, then it is likely that oestrogen was the cause. Very often there will be other pointers to hormonal sensitivity such as sensitivity to the Pill. If this is the case, you would be advised to consider a non-hormonal method of contraception and pay particular attention to your diet and exercise habits to counteract the fat storage encouraged by oestrogen.

If you started to take the Pill at an early age and simultaneously developed cellulite, this suggests a disturbance in the pituitary-ovarian axis, making the fatty tissues more sensitive to oestrogen. You need to limit exposure to further oestrogen by choosing a non-hormonal method of contraception. However, remember that despite all the problems associated with cellulite, none are as far-reaching as an unplanned pregnancy. So do discuss it fully with your doctor or health professional first. Often it is better to try every other means available to cure your cellulite and then if you really see no change after a few months, that is the time to stop taking the Pill.

If pregnancy was the precipitating factor, then there is less need for concern. Pregnancy is, after all, a temporary situation where you have a high oestrogen and calorie intake. After the birth, providing you take steps to clear yourself of cellulite, it should not recur unless you become pregnant again. Remember that breast-feeding is the only way to remove fat from the lower body after pregnancy. However, if you have had several pregnancies and gained weight after each one, it is necessary to look at the possibility of an iodine deficiency and consider taking iodine supplements to help get rid of the existing cellulite and prevent its reoccurrence.

If there does not seem to be any specific cause of your cellulite and it has just slowly crept on with the years, it could be due to a genetic susceptibility, particularly if there's a history of cellulite in your family. Absence of a family history of cellulite does not necessarily rule out genetic susceptibility, but do search a little more into your own health background and look carefully for any potential precipitating causes.

ARE THERE ANY OTHER CO-EXISTING FACTORS THAT NEED TREATMENT?

Any co-existing factors should be treated without hesitation

Do any of the following apply to you?

- Food allergies
- Constipation
- Poor posture or lordosis
- Smoking
- Poor diet
- Lack of exercise
- Sugar craving or hypoglycaemia

The above *must* be treated if you are to rid yourself of cellulite.

IS IT DYSMORPHISM?

Dysmorphism requires different treatment

Remember, treatment for dysmorphism, or "footballer's legs", needs a different approach. To assess whether you have dysmorphism, answer the following questions.

1 Look first at your body shape. Is your upper body slim, and are your legs muscular and much bigger in proportion to the upper body?

2 Are the fronts of your thighs bulkier than the rest of your legs? Do they appear heavy over the muscle area but not so much over the knees? Do the muscles seem to have a good covering of fatty tissue?

3 Do your thighs get noticeably bigger the more you exercise?

4 Do the thighs get smaller again after several weeks of not exercising?

5 Pinch the skin over your waist. Now pinch the skin over the front of your thighs. Is there a huge difference? Up to 1 or 2cm is normal, but a difference of over 2cm suggests a degree of dysmorphism.

If you answered "yes" to the above questions it is highly likely that you have dysmorphism. Untreated, it will simply get worse, particularly if you continue your existing exercise patterns. What you need, in this instance, is a balanced exercise regime that will work both the upper and lower body; one that focuses on building muscle on the upper body but not on the lower body. For example, you could work out using weights for the upper body and then do some gentle cycling for your legs, avoiding steep hills. If using an exercise bike, make sure it is on the "flat" or "gentle hills" setting. Or you could combine upper body weights work with dance or swimming. Stretching and weight-bearing exercise such as walking or dance will benefit both cellulite and dysmorphism.

In addition, you will need to pay attention to the microcirculation, so stop smoking, limit your caffeine intake and consider taking antioxidant vitamin and mineral supplements. If this does not help and you see no improvement, be prepared to seek professional help.

IS YOUR BODY IN THE BEST POSSIBLE SHAPE?

Taking good care of your body will ensure it maintains its natural harmony

If you are concerned about cellulite, no doubt you will be concerned about your overall body shape and weight. And whether you are thin or fat, if you suffer from cellulite your shape will be distorted. Although we cannot change our basic body shape, we can make the best of what we've got and improve it through diet and exercise.

BODY WEIGHT

Body weight is easy to measure, easy to record—and easy for doctors to nag about! The scales will give us our total body weight, but they will not differentiate between fat, fluid and muscle mass, which in fact are much more important.

Most of us have, from time to time, consulted the traditional height/weight tables to see if we fall into the "normal" range. However, since an underweight person can be troubled by cellulite just as much as an overweight person, merely losing weight so that you fall into the "normal" range will not resolve your cellulite problem.

Another way to assess if you are under- or overweight is to use the Body Mass Index (BMI), which expresses your weight in relation to your height. To calculate your BMI, first measure your height in metres and your weight in kilograms. Square your height (height x height), then divide your weight by your squared height. The resulting figure is your Body Mass Index. In other words: weight in kilograms/height x height in metres = BMI.

Any figure between 19 and 25 is considered a normal weight. Above this, and you are considered obese. Below this range and you are considered underweight, so in this instance a weight-reducing diet would not be suitable. Obesity is associated with many health risks, so if you are grossly overweight you obviously need to follow a suitable weight-reducing diet, regardless of any cellulite you may have. But for those who are comfortably in the middle, yet still have cellulite, this is of little help. And it still does not tell us how much fat, fluid and muscle mass we have. So what else can we do?

BODY MASS

The distribution of fat, fluid and muscle mass within the body gives us a far more accurate picture of our body size in relation to our health. Body fat, muscle and fluid content can be determined by measuring your weight, height and by using calipers to measure the thickness of the skin at certain points on the body. As it is difficult to take your own measurements—there is a skill in knowing exactly where to place the calipers—it's best to consult a professional. Many health clubs and gyms will automatically include this as part of a fitness assessment.

There are also sophisticated pieces of equipment that can assist in determining body composition which give a fairly accurate assessment, although the tried and tested skin thickness method is the most reliable.

Knowing whether we have too much fat, too much fluid or too little muscle mass will tell us whether we have an excess fat or water storage problem and can help us devise an appropriate exercise and diet routine to change the proportion of fat and muscle in the body.

THE MIRROR

The simplest technique for assessing our shape is—the mirror! By simply looking in the mirror we can see at a glance where we have too much fat and too little muscle.

The desire to have a well-proportioned body with a good shape will perhaps influence the success of our anti-cellulite campaign more than anything else. However, there is no such thing as "the perfect female shape"; every race has its specific build and shape and each culture its own ideal. But, in reality, what determines a good shape is down to the individual. So, we're back to where we started—in front of the mirror!

Having assessed your cellulite, the next step is to get rid of it. A healthy lifestyle with sensible eating and regular exercise is the best way to achieve a healthy body and prevent the occurrence of cellulite in the first place. And it is certainly the first step to take in ridding ourselves of existing cellulite. However, remember that once cellulite is well established, it is necessary to combine this with additional treatment, and in Part Two, we'll be looking at the various treatment methods available.

PART TWO:
THE TREATMENT

There must be hundreds of potential remedies for cellulite on the market—diets, creams, lotions and potions—many of them promising fantastic results in just a short period of time. So why do very few of them work?

First, it is important to understand that treatment for cellulite has to take the form of a systematic, *integrated* approach. As we now know, there are many causes of cellulite and, if untreated, these causes will continue to act and stimulate the further development of cellulite. Once it has formed, cellulite responds to each and every stimulus, even if that particular influence may have been at one time quite harmless. True, there may have been only one precipitating factor that set the whole avalanche in motion, but now we have to shift every flake of snow. *Every* possible factor has to be addressed, regardless of the original cause. It's not enough therefore simply to make changes to your diet and exercise regime, although this certainly should be the starting point. But such changes must be made in conjunction with other treatment techniques.

Second, you must accept that any treatment regime will take time to work. A simple cut takes a few days to heal, a bruise a week and a broken bone three to six weeks. These ailments heal well because the surrounding tissues have a good blood supply. However, since cellulite tissue has a poor blood supply, the healing process starts out with a major handicap. To treat cellulite effectively, we have to get the body to alter its cell structure through its own repairing mechanism, and that takes time. Furthermore, cellulite may have been present over a long period—ten to twenty years in many cases—and misguided attempts at treatment may have actually caused further damage.

Third, cellulite occupies a relatively large area of the body. Every square millimetre of affected tissue therefore has to be treated. As you can appreciate, this is a time-consuming process.

As we go step by step through the treatment schedule, remember that much of this is not only valid for dealing with existing cellulite but also for the prevention of further cellulite. Bearing in mind that some 95 per cent of women are likely to develop cellulite at some stage of their lives, taking care of our bodies should become second nature. Although cellulite cannot be cured through diet and exercise alone, a good diet and exercise regime is the foundation of any effective treatment programme. And not only will it help get rid of your cellulite, but it will also help you to a healthier, more active lifestyle. You will look and feel better and function more efficiently.

For those of you who are pregnant or who are considering having a child, remember that there is more and more evidence to show that many diseases may begin in the womb. This may also be true of cellulite—or at least the potential to develop cellulite. If you are already pregnant, you may not be able to follow all of the anti-cellulite measures included in this book, but eating a healthy diet and remaining active during pregnancy may well help protect your child from developing cellulite, or indeed many other diseases, in later life.

7

THE CELLULITE-CONTROL DIET

A good diet is the mainstay of any cellulite treatment

Although there is no single diet that will treat cellulite, a healthy and balanced eating plan forms a crucial part of any effective treatment regime. However, any change in your diet must take into account your lifestyle and the amount of calories and nutrients that you need during the course of the day, depending on your activity level. Whether or not you need to lose excess weight, following the step-by-step advice in this chapter will help you regulate your weight and get rid of unhealthy eating habits while ensuring a balanced intake of nutrients and ultimately helping you in your battle against cellulite. Some steps need to be taken in conjunction with others and this will be made clear in the text.

Don't set yourself unobtainable targets, but start by introducing changes gradually. Some changes may be more difficult than others, so you might want to adopt the easier ones first and then move on to the more difficult ones. Of course, this may slow down your progress, but the important thing is that you do make progress, however slowly, rather than give up altogether.

BEFORE YOU START

Before starting out on a new eating regime, first keep a record of everything you eat over a period of four days. There is no need to weigh each food, but just make a note of approximate quantities. Weighing everything you eat will only increase the likelihood of you altering your diet in this period so that you tend only to eat foods that are easy to weigh and therefore end up with a misleading result. Or, alternatively, you may simply become bored by the whole process and give up altogether.

Keeping a record of what you eat should tell you which foods form the basis of your existing diet as well as when and how much you eat and, perhaps, why you eat. Often, we don't just eat because we are hungry but also for comfort or out of boredom. Also, it is a known fact that we all underestimate the amount of food we eat. It is easy to forget that biscuit we had with the morning coffee or that bar of chocolate we devoured while waiting for the bus, so do make sure you keep an accurate record. This will enable you to see where the extra calories or junk foods have crept in. The frequency with which certain foods are eaten may also point to the possibility of a food allergy or intolerance.

STEP ONE: MINIMISE YOUR INTAKE OF ARTIFICIAL COLOURINGS, FLAVOURINGS AND ADDITIVES

Artificial colourings and additives can cause cellulite in sensitive individuals by interfering with the detoxifying enzyme system of the body. Artificial colourings are now known to cause hyperactivity in children. In adults, the changes may be more subtle such as water retention.

Such artificial products are found in a vast array of modern-day foods: pre-prepared foods, ready-made meals, tinned foods, instant products, cakes, puddings, pâtés, sausages, processed meats—the list is endless. The best way to avoid or at least cut down on your intake of artificial products is to prepare meals yourself using fresh ingredients. Instead of having a ready-made meal straight out of the freezer for supper, have a lean chop or fish with fresh vegetables, or even baked beans on toast. Don't think that your diet has to become bland or boring. With a little imagination and a good use of herbs, spices and dressings, you can create dishes that are equally good if not better and certainly healthier than any found on the supermarket shelves. Fresh meat, poultry, fish, vegetables, fruit and milk which should form the basis of your diet should not by law contain any added colourings.

A few additives are quite harmless as they are vitamins or food extracts and serve to prevent the food from deteriorating. The worst offenders in terms of chemical intolerance seem to be colourings and most preservatives. Additive antioxidants and emulsifiers are less troublesome, but it is still advisable to keep these to a minimum.

The following additives are derived from natural food substances and may be regarded as non-toxic in a cellulite-control diet.

Colours (E100–E180)

Avoid all but the following:

E100	curcumin
E101	riboflavin
E120	cochineal
E140	chlorophyll
E141	copper compounds of chlorophyll
E160a	carotene
E160b	annatto
E160c	capsanthin
E160d	lycopene
E160e	beta-apo-8'-carotenal
E160f	ethyl ester of beta-apo-8'-carotenal
E161	xanthophyll
E162	beetroot red
E163	anthocyanins
E170	calcium carbonate
E171	titanium dioxide
E172	iron oxides
E174	silver
E175	gold

Preservatives (E200–E299)

Avoid all but the following:

E200	sorbic acid
E201	sodium sorbate
E202	potassium sorbate
E203	calcium sorbate
E260	acetic acid
E290	carbon dioxide

Antioxidants (E300–E320)

Avoid all but the following:

E300	vitamin C
E301	vitamin C
E302	vitamin C
E304	ascorbyl palmitate
E306	vitamin E
E307	vitamin E
E308	vitamin E
E309	vitamin E

STEP TWO: REMOVE ARTIFICIAL SWEETENERS FROM YOUR DIET

Artificial sweeteners can have the same effect as chemical additives by overloading the body's detoxifying system and resulting in water retention. In sugar-sensitive individuals artificial sweeteners may also stimulate the release of insulin, thus causing water retention and weight gain.

Avoid products labelled "no added sugar," diet and low-calorie drinks since these will almost certainly contain some of the artificial sweeteners aspartame, acesulfame K, saccharin or sorbitol. It may not be easy at first, but in doing so, you will gently wean yourself off sweet things and re-educate your palate. Removing artificial sweeteners from your diet can lead to a weight loss of 1 or 2kg. This can be attributed to the loss of water previously retained by the inappropriate stimulation of insulin. The added bonus is that as you lose your sweet tooth, the desire for salty foods often disappears at the same time.

STEP THREE: CONTROL YOUR SODIUM INTAKE

Sodium (salt) in excess causes fluid retention in sensitive individuals. At present, there is no way of determining who has a susceptibility to sodium and who has not. However, a certain amount of sodium is necessary for normal water balance.

A blood test and a urine sodium measurement, which can be obtained through your GP, can detect if you have an adequate balance of sodium in the body. However, this is not necessary for most individuals, unless they are considering cellulite treatment by cellulolipolysis (a medical treatment where electrical currents are passed through the cellulite tissue) where the concentration of sodium in the body is important.

A regular intake of high-sodium foods can lead to excess sodium levels so avoid eating salty foods such as salt beef, smoked foods, processed foods, crisps and sprinkling liberal amounts of salt on your food. A simple rule of thumb is to add salt during cooking but not at the table. In hot weather, however, you can add extra salt to your food to compensate for the sodium lost through perspiration.

FOODS WITH A HIGH SODIUM CONTENT

Cut down on your intake of the following foods:

Anchovies
Bacon
Blue cheese
Crisps
Gammon
Feta cheese
Ham
Olives
Packeted savoury snacks
Pastrami

Prawns
Processed cheese
Processed meats
Salami
Salt Cod
Salted nuts
Smoked products (salmon, cod, haddock, meat)

STEP FOUR: ENSURE AN ADEQUATE BUT NOT EXCESSIVE INTAKE OF WATER

We all need a good intake of pure water such as mineral water or filtered tap water. However, if your cellulite has been caused through water retention, this means that the veins and lymph vessels are unable to adequately remove fluid from the tissues of the legs. Drinking excessive amounts of water can therefore exacerbate this problem.

As a rule of thumb, drink according to your thirst. Under normal conditions an intake of 1.5 litres per day is sufficient. In hot, dry environments this figure may rise to 3 litres per day and, of course, after exercise you will need to replenish water lost through perspiration. Let your thirst be the judge—not hearsay!

STEP FIVE: REMOVE EXCESS FAT FROM YOUR DIET

This step should be combined with exercise, suitable creams or medical treatment to remove fat from the cellulite areas

Removing excess fat from your diet will benefit your health in many ways and also aid weight loss.

A word of warning, however! Remember that in women fat is preferentially stored on the lower body and released from the upper body. Therefore, if you are embarking on a weight-reducing diet it is essential that you combine this with other forms of treatment such as exercise (see Chapter 9) and lipolytic aromatherapy mixtures or creams (see Chapter 10). In other words, mixtures and creams that encourage the removal of fat from the area to which they are applied. Otherwise fat will tend to remain on the lower body at the expense of fat stores on the upper body. If the above measures have been taken and no further improvement is seen, it may be that medical intervention by mesotherapy and cellulolipolysis is necessary.

A certain amount of fat in your food is important for health but this should come from vegetable and fish sources, not animal sources. A small amount of fat also slows down digestion, allowing you to feel full for longer and avoid those peckish moments. Certain fats which are essential for the normal functioning of the body are unable to be manufactured by the body itself. These fats are known as essential fatty acids and are found in vegetable sources such as wheatgerm and vegetable oils such as sunflower, safflower, sesame, walnut and grapeseed oil. Other fats found in fish oils are known as eicosapaentanoic acids—or EPA for short— and protect against heart disease and other degenerative conditions. Because of their anti-inflammatory nature and the protection they offer to the small blood vessels, they may even prove to help prevent cellulite.

Certain conditions, such as eczema and dry or irritated skin, benefit, not from a high-fat diet, but from a diet rich in essential fatty acids. The three essential fatty acids are linoleic acid, alpha linolenic acid and gamma linolenic or GLA. They can be obtained in a high concentration from evening primrose oil, starflower (borage) oil and safflower oil capsules, available from most chemists and health food stores. If in doubt about your need for essential fatty acids, check with your doctor.

In our anti-cellulite regime what we want to achieve is a reduction in the total amount of fat in the diet, which will automatically lead to a reduction in the proportion of calories obtained from fat. The remaining calories in our diet should be derived from carbohydrates, fruit and protein. The amount of these that we need each day will depend on our individual energy requirements.

To cut down on the fat in our diet, it is not just a question of reducing our intake of all visible fats such as butter, cream and oils or by trimming fat off meat. There are many hidden sources of fat in foods such as chocolate, cakes and biscuits. Chocolate is 50 per cent fat, so the next time you munch on a bar, remember that half of it is fat. The other half, by the way, is mostly sugar!

Although frying is not encouraged as a means of cooking, it is acceptable to lightly fry certain foods such as white fish, chicken and calf's liver since these foods are already low in fat. Use only vegetable oil and use as little as possible. Dab the food with a kitchen towel after frying to remove all traces of fat. It is wise not to choose to eat fried foods in restaurants and in takeaway meals where you have no control over the amount of fat used in the cooking.

Check out the following list which contains foods too high in fat to be of value in a cellulite-control diet.

FOODS TO AVOID

Biscuits, chocolate, cakes and pastries

Just about all these foods are high in fat and/or sugar
Marzipan should also be avoided

Butter and oils

All oils except safflower, sunflower, walnut, grapeseed and
　　sesame oil (keep consumption to a minimum)
Butter
Ghee
Lard
Margarine

Eggs

Fried eggs
Omelettes
Pancakes
Scotch eggs

Fish

Any fish tinned in oil (choose fish tinned in water or brine)
Fish fried in batter
Fish roe
Herring: raw, cooked, pickled
Kippers
Sardines
Sprats
Taramasalata
Whitebait

Meat, poultry and meat products

Bacon rashers
Beefburgers (unless made from lean meat)
High-fat mince (choose lean or extra lean)
Liver sausage
Luncheon meat
Meat with visible fat (trim fat off)
Pâté

Pork belly rashers
Pork pies
Pork spare ribs
Poultry with skin (remove skin before cooking)
Salami
Sausages
Sausage rolls
Tongue

Milk and milk products

All hard and soft cheeses except cottage cheese and low-fat
   cheese
Cheesecake
Cream
Cream cheese
Full-fat milk (choose skimmed or semi-skimmed)

Nuts

All nuts (except chestnuts) and nut products, for example, peanut
butter, tahini, hummus

Savoury snacks

Just about all these products are high in fat; for example, crack-
   ers, crisps, savoury sticks and snacks, poppadoms, bhajees

Miscellaneous

Avocado and avocado-based dips and spreads, for example,
   guacamole

STEP SIX: REDUCE YOUR SUGAR INTAKE

*This step should be combined with the use of cellulite creams,
exercise or medical techniques. Nutritional supplements may
also be necessary.*

Sugar in the diet is stored in the liver as glycogen. When these
stores are full, any excess sugar is stored as fat, again preferentially
on the lower body. However, since the body prefers to use sugar
rather than fat for the production of energy, sugar can be more
rapidly burnt off.

Sugars are carbohydrates. Broadly speaking, carbohydrates split into two main groups: simple carbohydrates (sugar) and complex carbohydrates (starches). Simple carbohydrates such as glucose and fructose are easily absorbed by the body and used for energy. In general, the more complex the sugar, the more slowly the sugar is digested, leading to a more gradual release of energy. This is why complex carbohydrates such as the starch found in potatoes, rice and pasta are far more useful than simple carbohydrates as an energy source for everyday and sporting activities. Because complex carbohydrates are digested more slowly than simple carbohydrates, the blood sugar level does not rise so rapidly. The insulin response is therefore tempered and the sugar is gradually burnt off throughout the course of the day.

Purists will argue that potatoes, white rice, refined pasta and white bread are not true complex carbohydrates and that they behave like simple carbohydrates. It is true that there are even more complex forms of carbohydrate which release their sugar extremely slowly over the course of the day. Unrefined cereals, wholemeal bread, brown rice, beans, lentils and other pulses are extremely complex carbohydrates with a high fibre content. These foods keep the sugar level very stable and also decrease the rate at which fat is absorbed; they are therefore excellent as part of an anti-cellulite regime. Very active people who need to maintain an adequate energy intake should aim to eat considerable amounts of these high-fibre foods rather than relying on a high-calorie snack to fill the gap, which is not recommended in the treatment of cellulite. However, it's not always easy or practical to live on beans and more beans in today's busy lifestyle! If you can, so much the better, particularly if your cellulite is troublesome. It is probably easier to consider such foods as being less complex carbohydrates, leaving the term complex carbohydrates to describe brown or unrefined pasta, rice, flour, whole cereals and bread products. Don't rely entirely on these more refined, less complex carbohydrates, aim to include some of the more complex products in your diet.

Simple sugars should be reduced to an absolute minimum in the diet and replaced by complex carbohydrates such as brown bread, rice, pasta, potatoes, beans and pulses. The amount of these foods that you need will depend on how active you are. It's a good idea to eat a high-carbohydrate breakfast such as cereals and milk, porridge, rehydrated dried fruits or toast and spread. See the sample diet section on pg. 97. This gives you instant energy so that the sugar released will be burnt up during the course of the day. Certain supplements such as glucose tolerance factor and zinc-nickel-cobalt oligosol (see Chapter 8) can help reduce sugar cravings.

If you need to lose weight, you will have to reduce your calorie intake accordingly or increase your level of activity—or both. If the fat is to be successfully burnt up, then the body's energy intake must be slightly less than its energy output so that the fat stores are gradually used up. But only slightly less—this has to be a gradual process if we are to maintain the fat stores on the upper body and keep the same bra size! Reducing your sugar intake will help reduce the absorption of fat, but remember, it's important also to combine this step with exercise and the use of a lipolytic cream to encourage the removal of fat from the lower body.

Many women with cellulite are not overweight and do not need or want to lose weight. They simply need to redistribute it. This can be achieved effectively through exercise and by altering the components of the diet (see step eleven).

The following list contains foods that are too high in sugar to be of value in a cellulite-control diet.

FOODS TO AVOID

Cakes, biscuits, pastries

Just about all these products are very high in sugar (and fat). Only savoury water biscuits and crispbreads are recommended.

Desserts

Ice cream
Milk-based puddings
Pies
Puddings
Sorbets
Tarts
Tinned fruit

Dried fruits

All foods containing dried fruit, for example, fruit cake, muesli
Apricots
Bananas
Currants
Dates
Figs

Mangoes
Peaches
Pears
Raisins
Sultanas

STEP SEVEN: CURTAIL YOUR ALCOHOL INTAKE

Alcohol improves blood supply by opening up the arteries and can also aid relaxation. Red wine contains tannins which protect and strengthen the microcirculation against damage from free radicals and therefore, in moderate doses, is beneficial in the treatment of cellulite. However, alcohol contains many calories which are rapidly turned to fat. In order to enjoy the benefits of alcohol but avoid the pitfalls, stick to one glass of wine, preferably red, per day.

STEP EIGHT: LIMIT YOUR COFFEE INTAKE

Caffeine in coffee and, to a lesser extent, in tea increases the basal metabolic rate—the rate at which we burn calories. In high doses, however, it causes a narrowing of the small blood vessels and it thus promotes cellulite. Your daily intake of caffeine should therefore be restricted to a maximum of three cups of instant coffee (one teaspoon per cup), two filter coffees or one expresso or cappuccino. Tea contains beneficial tannins and far less caffeine than coffee so you need not concern yourself with its restriction. Remember that too much tea can cause constipation, so be careful if you are prone to that particular problem. Also pay attention to the amount of liquid contained in the tea—see step 4, page 75.

STEP NINE: INCLUDE PLENTY OF FRESH VEGETABLES IN YOUR DIET

Vegetables and salads add bulk to your diet and contain valuable vitamins, minerals and essential oils that help repair cellulite tissue. Vegetables, particularly the brightly coloured ones such as tomatoes, red peppers and spinach, are rich in important antioxidant vitamins and minerals which protect the small blood vessels against damage from free radicals and therefore play an important role in an anti-cellulite regime.

In order to maximise their vitamin potential, store vegetables in a cool place, away from heat and sunlight and eat them as fresh as possible. Cooking vegetables tends to decrease their vitamin content so, wherever possible, eat them raw or cook for the minimum amount of time in a small amount of water. Steaming or microwaving also reduces the loss of vitamins and helps retain flavour.

Raw foods such as fruit and vegetables contain valuable enzymes and plant hormones that play an important role in maintaining the healthy functioning of the body and also help detoxify artificial food products. Furthermore, raw foods contain a certain electromagnetic energy which is destroyed in the cooking and storing process. Suffice it to say that raw food should form a reasonable proportion of your diet.

Some vegetables and vegetable extracts are commonly used in the treatment of medical disorders, especially on the Continent. For instance, carrot juice is used to treat digestive problems, potato juice to treat ulcers and cabbage juice to treat gastritis.

The following vegetables also contain specific properties that are useful in the treatment of cellulite.

Artichoke stimulates the liver to remove toxins held within. It also aids the passage of faeces through the intestines and stimulates the removal of fat from fat cells.
Seaweed contains iodine which stimulates the thyroid gland. The thyroid gland controls the metabolic rate, and a deficiency in iodine can therefore slow down the rate at which we burn calories.
Nettles, for instance in herbal teas, stimulate the kidneys, thus helping remove excess fluid from the body.
Garlic is a powerful anti-cholesterol agent and protects the small blood vessels from damage. It also improves the blood supply to all tissues in the body, including the fatty tissues.

RECOMMENDED VEGETABLES

Eat as wide a selection of vegetables as possible.

Vegetable	*Health benefit*
Asparagus	Contains some vitamin C and beta-carotene
Bamboo shoots	Rich in silica, which improves circulation
Beans, French, runner, string	Contains some beta-carotene and other vitamins

Vegetable	Health benefit
Beansprouts	Contains valuable enzymes for digestion and wellbeing
Broccoli	Rich in beta-carotene and vitamin C
Brussels sprouts	Contains some beta-carotene and vitamin C
Cabbage	Rich in iron, vitamin C, beta-carotene and fibre
Carrots	Rich in beta-carotene
Cauliflower	Contains some vitamins and minerals
Celery	Contains some vitamins and minerals; diuretic
Chicory/endive	High in folic acid (essential vitamin)
Chinese leaves	Contains some vitamins and minerals
Courgettes	Contains some vitamins and minerals
Fennel	Aids digestion and stabilises sugar level if eaten raw
Globe artichoke	Aids passage of faeces through intestines; stimulates liver and removes liver toxins; aids fat-burning process; diuretic
Kale	Rich in iron, vitamin C, beta-carotene and fibre
Leeks	Rich in mucilage (aids bowel transit); aids bowel flora
Mange-tout	Rich in vitamin C
Mushrooms	Rich in vitamin B5 for healthy skin and hair
Okra	Rich in mucilage; aids bowel function; rich in folic acid

Vegetable	*Health benefit*
Onions	Rich in mucilage; stimulates bowel flora; rich in sulphur for healthy skin
Peas	High in protein; rich in vitamin C and fibre
Peppers, red and green	Very rich in beta-carotene, vitamin C and flavonoids for free radical protection
Spinach	Rich in iron, beta-carotene and fibre
Squash	Contains some vitamins and minerals
Tomatoes	Very rich in beta-carotene, vitamin C, flavonoids
Watercress	Very rich in beta-carotene, vitamin C, flavonoids, sulphur protein and fibre.

STEP TEN: SEPARATE FRUIT FROM MEALS

Although fruit is an excellent source of vitamins, fibre, minerals and trace elements, some fruits are rich in sugar. The sugar is present as fructose, a fruit sugar which although natural is nevertheless sugar and still generates calories. Fructose is easily absorbed by the body and, like other sugars, may increase the absorption of fat from the diet if eaten simultaneously.

The amount of sugar present varies according to the specific fruit. For instance, bananas contain mostly starch and insufficient vitamins to be of use in an anti-cellulite diet, while blackcurrants, strawberries, blueberries and other soft fruits contain little sugar and are also rich in the antioxidant vitamin C, which makes them an excellent choice when treating cellulite.

Whatever its sugar content, *fruit should always be eaten separately from meals*. Allow at least two hours between eating fruit and a meal. This will prevent the sugar-fat absorption system from taking place as well as aiding digestion.

Dried fruits also contain natural sugar and are very high in calories. Eaten dry as pick-me-up snacks and nibbles they are too rich

or an anti-cellulite regime and should generally be avoided.
However, since dried fruits contain high levels of calcium, iron,
fibre and minerals, providing they are soaked overnight in water,
they may be eaten at breakfast time so that the sugar can be burned
off by the body during the course of the day.

FRUITS RELATIVELY HIGH IN SUGAR

Limit your intake of these to 225g (8oz) per day:

Bananas
Blueberries
Dried apricots stewed in water
Grapes, black
Grapes, white
Lychees
Mangoes

FRUITS WITH A FAIR AMOUNT OF SUGAR

Limit your intake to 450g (1lb) per day:

Cherries
Pineapple

FRUITS WITH LITTLE SUGAR

Can be eaten in unlimited quantities:

Apples	Melon
Apricots	Nectarines
Bilberries	Papaya
Blackberries	Peaches
Blackcurrants	Pears
Figs	Plums
Gooseberries	Raspberries
Grapefruit	Strawberries
Loganberries	Tangerines

STEP ELEVEN: FOLLOW THE FOOD-COMBINING AND SEPARATION PRINCIPLES

Although medical research has yet to prove or disprove the facts,
there is no doubt that many people have found a food-combining
diet to be of enormous benefit in the treatment of a number of complaints ranging from digestive problems to chronic fatigue and cel-

lulite. In fact, the term "food separation" is perhaps more accurate as the principle of this type of diet is that you separate proteins and starches so that they are never eaten together in the same meal. This enables the body's digestive system to function more efficiently.

The reason for this is that proteins and starches require different sets of enzymes in order to be properly digested. Protein-digesting enzymes prefer to work in an acid environment, while starch-digesting enzymes prefer an alkaline environment. If the two are forced to work together, neither is working in its preferred environment and, consequently, neither is functioning at optimum efficiency.

In fact, our digestive system was simply not designed to cope with an influx of different food products all in one go. If we look back in the evolutionary process to ancient times, we know that man was a hunter-gatherer who hunted small mammals and gathered nuts and berries. Just imagine what it was like living wild in the forest. You are hungry, so you hunt and catch, say, a bird and eat it. Later that day you are hungry again, so you go in search of more food. Birds are not easy to catch so instead you find a bush full of blackberries and eat your fill. You are now full and the day is over. The next day you will again eat what you can find, perhaps some nuts, maybe a tuber that you can uproot, or even some more berries.

Get the picture? Ancient man did not sit down each day to meat and two veg but satisfied his hunger with just one or two basic foods. He was, in effect, a "food separator." Of course, he had no choice. But these days we have more than enough choices and our diet has become more and more complex.

Of course, there are people who can eat anything and not suffer any ill-effects, just as there are smokers who smoke all their lives and have never had a coughing fit in the morning. We all know people who are exceptions to the rule. The point is, however, that everyone has a threshold, depending on their body's ability to counteract any damage, and once we pass that threshold we will develop certain symptoms. Those with a low threshold will be sensitive to certain stimuli. Cellulite is all about sensitivity to various stimuli and diet is just one of these.

THE FOOD-COMBINING PRINCIPLES

The bulk of the diet should be made up of protein, carbohydrate (starches and sugars), fruit and vegetables. The general principle is not to eat protein in the same meal as carbohydrate.

- **Protein** may be eaten with vegetables and pulses, but *not* carbohydrates (starches and sugars) or fruit.
- **Carbohydrates** (starches and sugars) may be eaten with vegetables and pulses, but *not* with protein.
- **Fruit and fruit juice** should be eaten separately from meals, with a gap of two hours in between.
- **Skimmed, semi-skimmed and low-fat milk and natural yoghurt** may be consumed with either proteins or starches, sugars, fruit and vegetables.

FOOD GROUPS AND COMBINATIONS

You may combine foods from any same vertical column to make up your meal, but you must not combine foods from different columns.

Protein	*Carbohydrates*	*Fruit*
Lamb	Rice	All fruits
Beef	Cereals	
Pork	Bread	
Chicken	Couscous	
Duck	Noodles	
Game	Pasta	
Turkey	Semolina	
Offal	Potatoes	
Fish	Polenta	
Shellfish	Buckwheat	
Eggs	Millet	
Cheese	Oats	
	Porridge	
	Cassava (gari)	
	Eddoes, yams	
	Plantains	
Pulses	Pulses	
Milk	Milk	
Yoghurt	Yoghurt	
(Salad and vegetables)	(Salad and vegetables)	(Salad and vegetables)

VALUE OF PROTEIN IN A CELLULITE-CONTROL DIET

Protein is important for tissue growth and repair, which is something we want to encourage in our battle against cellulite. We also need adequate protein in the diet to help us build lean muscle tissue as we tone up in our exercise campaign. Excess protein in the diet is ultimately converted to carbohydrate by means of a complex and time-consuming process that ensures the body has a slow-release source of energy to fall back on.

Protein also stimulates the basal metabolic rate, generating heat and burning calories. A decent steak acts as a better pick-me-up for a cold and hungry person than any amount of starch. It also lasts longer and provides protein as well as calories that will not rapidly turn into fat. Meat, fish, poultry, eggs, milk and yoghurt are all rich sources of protein.

FOODS ALLOWED ON A CELLULITE-CONTROL DIET

The following lists contain foods that are permissable in a cellulite-control diet. Suggested cooking methods are given, but these are by no means exhaustive. So be adventurous and experiment with different flavours—without adding fat! Add lemon juice, herbs and spices for extra taste and variety.

RECOMMENDED PROTEIN DISHES

Can be combined with vegetables, pulses and fat (limit the fat!)

Beef:
Minced beef, made into beef
   burgers and grilled
Lean mince, dry-fried
Minute steak, stir-fried with sauces
Roast, no fat, serve hot or cold
Steak, grilled or made into kebabs

Chicken:
Breast, roasted, casseroled or
   microwaved, serve hot or cold
Roast, no fat or skin
Thighs, roasted, casseroled or
   microwaved, serve hot or cold

Dairy products: Milk (preferably skimmed,
    semi-skimmed or low-fat)*
Cheese (low-fat)
Cottage cheese
Quark
Yoghurt (low-fat, no added sugar)*

Duck: Breast, roasted, no fat

Eggs: Boiled
En Cocotte
Poached

Fish: All the following can be barbecued,
    grilled, poached, smoked (in moderation) or
    lightly fried (remove oil after cooking).
Tinned fish (in brine or water) is
    also permissible.

Any white or flat fish:
Carp
Cod
Coley
Conger
Haddock
Hake
Halibut
Monkfish
Plaice
Rock salmon
Salmon
Shark
Skate
Sole
Swordfish
Tilapia
Trout
Tuna
Whiting

See note under Extras

Game:
: All the following are low in fat and may be roasted, casseroled, microwaved or stewed:

  Guinea fowl
  Hare
  Partridge
  Pheasant
  Quail
  Rabbit

Lamb:
: Chops, grilled, trim off visible fat
  Lean mince
  Leg steaks, braised with lemon juice and herbs
  Leg, roast, no fat
  Neck fillet, make into kebabs
  Noisettes, grilled

Miscellaneous:
: Quorn

Offal:
: Kidney, casseroled, lightly fried (remove oil after cooking) or make into kebabs and barbecue or grill
  Liver, casseroled or lightly fried (remove oil after cooking)

Pork:
: Chops, grilled, trim off visible fat
  Fillet, grilled, casseroled or cooked in sweet and sour sauce
  Kebabs, grilled or barbecued
  Lean mince

Pulses:
: Beans:
  Aduki
  Blackeye
  Borlotti
  Flageolet
  Haricot
  Mung
  Red Kidney
  Soya

Peas:
> Chickpeas
> Dahl
> Green peas
> Hummus (check fat content,
> many preparations include too
> much oil)
> Lentils
> Split peas
> Yellow peas

Seafood:
All the following can be boiled,
> grilled, barbecued and served hot or cold
> with low-calorie dressing if desired:
>> Mussels
>> Prawns, king prawns, tiger prawns
>> Octopus
>> Shrimps
>> Squid

Soya products:
Miso
Tofu
TVP
Vegetable burgers (made with
soya)

Turkey:
Grilled, casseroled, microwaved
Kebabs, barbecued or grilled
Lean mince
Roasted with skin removed

RECOMMENDED CARBOHYDRATE (STARCH) DISHES

Can be combined with vegetables and pulses

Where possible, choose wholemeal bread, pasta, rice and noodles
in preference to refined carbohydrates.

Baked beans: on toast, with jacket potatoes
Buckwheat: roast buckwheat kernels, spaghetti
with vegetable or tomato dressing
Noodles: with vegetable dressings and sauces,
Chinese vegetables, herbs

Pasta:	with vegetable sauce, tomato sauce, herbs (for example, basil), beans, salad
Polenta:	with tomatoes, mushrooms, peppers and other vegetables
Potatoes:	baked in jackets and served with low-calorie spread or low-calorie mayonnaise or boiled and served with low-calorie margarine or low-calorie mayonnaise
Rice:	with vegetables, tomatoes, peas, beans, corn

PULSES

Although pulses contain protein, they are regarded as neutral, in which case they can be eaten or mixed with either protein or carbohydrate, but not both in the same meal. If mixed with protein *or* carbohydrate, then they will be classed accordingly.

VEGETABLES AND SALADS

Vegetables and vegetable juices include all green and coloured vegetables and mushrooms, and these may be eaten at any time with all food groups.

Potatoes, yams, sweet potatoes and corn on the cob are considered as carbohydrates and therefore must not be eaten with protein.

EXTRAS

Although they contain protein, yoghurt and milk can be eaten with any food group. Chose natural or bio yoghurt, low-fat if possible, and skimmed or semi-skimmed milk.

PUTTING IT ALL TOGETHER

Now that you know what you can eat and which foods can be combined in a meal, you need to know how much of each food group you can eat for a balanced diet. Remember that your calorie intake should not exceed your energy output if you are to maintain your existing weight. However, if you need to lose weight, you either need to eat fewer calories or increase your level of activity or both.

YOUR WEEKLY EATING PLAN

HOW MUCH PROTEIN AND CARBOHYDRATE?

We all need a certain amount of protein for muscle building, tissue repair and general health, and we also need sufficient carbohydrates for energy and to help the protein to do its rebuilding and repairing job. Any unwanted protein can be converted to carbohydrate by the body, so it's never wasted. As this conversion process requires a little time and energy on the body's part, generally protein does not contribute to the fat-storing process in the same way as carbohydrate and sugar.

The relative amounts of protein and carbohydrate we need depend on the amount of activity we undertake. Broadly speaking, this can be divided into three different groups: not very active; fairly active; and very active. Choose the group that matches your activity levels and follow the guidelines on page 96.

Excluding breakfast, there are fourteen meals (lunches and evening meals) per week. Breakfast remains free because the digestive system is working at its peak first thing in the morning so you can break the food-combining rules here and choose from cereal and milk, toast, reduced-sugar jam, porridge or yoghurt.

Fruit may be eaten between meals providing you allow a two-hour gap before eating a meal. For the remainder of your meals use the guidelines below. Remember to include plenty of vegetables with both carbohydrate and protein meals. When choosing your meals, don't forget to avoid excess sugar and fat. Use fresh ingredients wherever possible and cut down on ready-made meals and takeaways. Low-fat yoghurt and skimmed or semi-skimmed milk can be taken with or between meals.

ADDITIONAL NOTES FOR VEGETARIANS

There are different types of "vegetarians." True vegetarians do not eat meat or fish, usually for moral reasons. But an increasing number of people are "demi-vegetarians" in that they have vegetarian-based diets that also include fish, eggs and sometimes chicken. Most vegetarians eat eggs, milk, milk products, yoghurt and cheese. Vegans, however, do not eat any animal products, including eggs, milk, cheese and milk products.

Most diets, if well balanced, can supply the body with all the essential nutrients. The main problem for vegetarians, especially vegans, is to include sufficient calcium, iron and vitamin B12 since these nutrients are derived mainly from meat and animal products. However, with a bit of careful planning, it is possible to include these nutrients in a vegetarian, cellulite-control diet.

Protein intake can also pose a problem for vegetarians. Fish and chicken are rich sources of protein, so "demi-vegetarians" or non-red-meat-eaters should not have any problem in terms of protein intake. True vegetarians, however, tend to obtain their protein from eggs, milk and milk products such as cheese which all have a fairly high fat content. Nuts and nut products, which are equally fatty, also form a large proportion of the vegetarian diet. Likewise, pre-prepared vegetarian dishes tend to be quite high in fat. Obviously, in an anti-cellulite regime, we need to limit our fat intake and ensure a good intake of nutrients and protein, so vegetarians need some extra help in planning their diet.

The following are low-fat, high-protein alternatives to cheese and nuts.

Quorn is a relatively new arrival in the supermarket and is prepared from certain fungi. It is high in protein and fibre but contains very little fat or carbohydrate. Quorn requires little preparation as it is sold in a ready-to-cook form. It has a pleasant nutty/meaty taste with a good texture but is slightly dry, so it is best cooked in a sauce. Quorn can be eaten on its own or with other foods such as pulses, eggs, low-fat cheese, yoghurt and soya products. It is classed as a protein food in our anti-cellulite regime.

Tofu is soya bean curd and comes in creamy white chunks. Again, it is high in protein and low in fat and so makes an ideal protein choice. It has a rather bland flavour and can be eaten on its own or with a tasty sauce or incorporated into dishes with eggs, milk, yoghurt, low-fat cheese or Quorn.

TVP or Textured Vegetable Protein is a processed soya flour. It forms the basis of most vegetable burgers, pre-prepared vegetarian meals and meat substitutes. Again it is classed as a protein food in our anti-cellulite regime.

Pulses include dried beans, lentils and peas and, nowadays, there are many tasty varieties available. With the exception of soya beans, pulses alone cannot provide the necessary amount of protein in the diet and therefore must be combined with other protein-rich foods. Pulses can be classed as either carbohydrate foods (and therefore mixed with grains), or proteins (and mixed with Quorn, soya, eggs, low-fat soft cheese, TVP and tofu).

Grains include wheat, bulghur, bread, pasta, barley, buckwheat, corn, couscous, millet, oats, rye and spelt (ancient strain of wheat). They are classed as carbohydrates. However, they do contain some protein, which is important in a vegetarian or vegan diet. They may be mixed with pulses to increase the amount of protein in the diet, yet at the same time they provide energy in the form of carbohydrates.

CHECKLIST OF NUTRIENTS FOR VEGETARIANS AND VEGANS

If you are a strict vegetarian or vegan, ensure that you have a good intake of the following nutrients which may be lacking in a typical vegetarian or vegan diet. It may be that you will need extra help in the form of a supplement.

Nutrient	Source
Vitamin B	Wholegrain cereals; wholemeal bread; green vegetables; wheatgerm; yeast extract; vitamin B supplements
Vitamin B12	Yeast extract; vitamin B12 supplements
Vitamin D	Margarine; fortified soya milk; eggs (if eaten); sunlight on the skin is also a source
Iron	Pulses; eggs (if eaten); wheatgerm; green vegetables; cocoa; molasses; dried fruits; iron supplements if necessary; vitamin C increases the absorption of iron
Calcium	Calcium-enriched soya milk; millet; dried fruits; hard water; calcium supplements

BREAKFAST

Aim to eat a satisfying breakfast to set you up for the rest of the morning so that you avoid high-calorie mid-morning snacks. Breakfast is the time to get your "fix" of sweet things and treats as you will burn off the calories during the course of the day.

Choose from:

Cereal with skimmed or semi-skimmed milk

Cereal with fruit
Porridge made with skimmed milk
Bananas
Non-sweet biscuits, crispbreads, water biscuits, oatcakes
Toast and reduced-sugar jam
Low-fat yoghurt

BETWEEN-MEAL SNACKS

Fruit (remember the limits and separate from meals)
Low-fat yoghurt
Vegetables

LUNCHES AND EVENING MEALS

GROUP 1: NOT VERY ACTIVE

Some people are not able to exercise due to injury, age or illness.
  Aim: Eat *twelve* protein-based meals and *two* carbohydrate-based meals per week in addition to breakfast.

GROUP 2: FAIRLY ACTIVE

Most of us, hopefully, fit into this group. It includes people who do a reasonable amount of exercise each week. This includes those who follow a formal exercise programme or who do the equivalent of an hour's walking each day or those people whose job involves a fair amount of activity.
  Aim: Eat *ten* protein-based meals and *four* carbohydrate-based meals in addition to breakfast. Ideally the carbohydrate-based meals should be taken on the day of exercise so that you have a ready store of energy.

GROUP 3: VERY ACTIVE

This group includes fitness instructors, dance teachers, PE instructors and other people who exercise in the course of their work or who have very active jobs or perform heavy physical tasks.
  Aim: Eat *seven* or *eight* protein-based meals and *six* or *seven* carbohydrate-based meals per week in addition to breakfast.

SAMPLE MENUS

WEEKDAY MENU 1

Carbohydrate snack lunch; protein evening meal. Useful for those who have a busy schedule during the day. Also ideal on exercise days.

Breakfast	Freshly squeezed orange juice Wholemeal toast with low-fat spread and reduced-sugar jam Coffee, tea or herbal tea (no sugar)
Mid-morning	Tea, herbal tea or water Apple
Lunch	Baked jacket potato with baked beans or low-calorie mayonnaise filling (home-made or takeaway) Low-fat yoghurt Herbal tea
Mid-afternoon	Tea, herbal tea or water Pear
Tea-time or on arrival at home	Tea, herbal tea or water Soft fruit; for example, melon, strawberries
Evening meal	Kebabs made from lamb fillets, beef steak, chicken or turkey flesh and peppers, onions and tomatoes (use garlic and herbs for flavour) with salad or vegetables

WEEKDAY MENU 2

Protein cooked lunch and evening meal

Breakfast	Freshly squeezed fruit juice
	Cereal with skimmed or semi-skimmed milk or low-fat yoghurt
	Coffee, tea or herbal tea (no sugar)
Mid-morning	Tea, herbal tea or water
	Apple
Lunch	Tomato, mushroom or vegetable soup
	Roast pork, beef or chicken with vegetables
	Low-fat yoghurt
Mid-afternoon	Tea, herbal tea or water
	Pear
Tea-time or on arrival at home	Tea, herbal tea or water
	Soft fruit; for example, melon, blueberries
Evening meal	Grilled salmon with salad

WEEKDAY MENU 3

Protein packed lunch; takeaway protein evening meal. Ideal for exercise days.

Breakfast
: Freshly squeezed orange juice
Porridge
Coffee, tea or herbal tea (no sugar)

Mid-morning
: Tea, herbal tea or water
Apple

Lunch
: Cold roast leg or breast of chicken
with tomatoes and peppers
Low-fat yoghurt

Mid-afternoon
: Tea, herbal tea or water
Orange

Tea-time or on arrival at home
: Two to three non-sweet biscuits if
exercising later

Evening meal
: Takeaway Chinese meal:
Soup (meat and/or vegetable
soup)
Meat, chicken or fish in sauce
but no rice
Vegetables or salad (steamed
or prepared at home if possible)
One glass wine if desired

WEEKDAY MENU 4

Protein restaurant lunch; protein evening meal

Breakfast	Freshly squeezed orange juice Stewed dried fruit: apricots, prunes or peaches Coffee, tea or herbal tea (no sugar)
Mid-morning	Tea, herbal tea or water Apple
Restaurant	Tomato juice, kir or one glass white wine as lunch aperitif Vegetable soup Choose from meat, fish, poultry, shellfish, lobster or crab (grilled, microwaved or poached) with vegetables and/or salad with French dressing One glass wine with main course (or two if aperitif not taken) Coffee or tea (no sugar)
Mid-afternoon	Tea, herbal tea or water Peach or nectarine
Tea-time or on arrival at home	Vegetable crudités with yoghurt dip or home-made vinaigrette dressing
Evening meal	Grilled fish or chicken with salad or vegetables

WEEKEND MENU 1

Carbohydrate lunch; protein evening meal

Breakfast	Fresh fruit salad Toast with low-fat spread or reduced-sugar jam Coffee, tea or herbal tea (no sugar)
Mid-morning	Tea, herbal tea or water Fruit
Lunch	Baked beans on toast Salad or vegetables
Mid-afternoon	Tea, herbal tea or water Fruit

Evening meal	Vegetable or meat soup
	Grilled steak with salad or
	    vegetables
	Low-fat yoghurt
	Two glasses wine (preferably red)
	    maximum

WEEKEND MENU 2

Roast Sunday lunch; carbohydrate evening meal

Breakfast   Fresh fruit salad
                           Toast with low-fat spread or reduced-
                              sugar jam
                           Coffee, tea or herbal tea (no
                              sugar)

Mid-morning   Fruit juice

Lunch   Smoked salmon, or prawns in low-fat
                              mayonnaise
                           Roast beef, lamb, pork, turkey or
                              chicken with gravy made from meat
                              juices (all fat removed), roast high-
                              protein sausages, roast mushrooms,
                              vegetables (no roast potatoes or roast
                              parsnips) or salad
                           Low-fat fromage frais
                           One glass wine (preferably red)

Mid-afternoon   Tea, herbal tea or water
                           Plums

Evening meal   Polenta with tomato and mushroom
                              topping
                           Low-fat yoghurt

VEGETARIAN MENU 1

Carbohydrate cooked lunch; protein evening meal

Breakfast	Fruit salad with low-fat fromage frais or low-fat cheese
	Coffee, tea or herbal tea (no sugar)
Mid-morning	Tea, herbal tea or water
	Apple
Lunch	Pasta with vegetable sauce and salad
Mid-afternoon	Tea, herbal tea or water
	Low-fat yoghurt
Tea-time or on arrival at home	One slice toast with low-fat spread or reduced-sugar jam
Evening meal	Bean casserole, tofu, tomatoes and vegetables

VEGETARIAN MENU 2

Carbohydrate lunch; protein evening meal

Breakfast	Fresh orange juice One slice toast with low-fat spread or reduced-sugar jam Coffee, tea or herbal tea (no sugar)
Mid-morning	Tea, herbal tea or water Piece of fruit
Lunch	Jacket potato with baked bean filling Tomato salad
Mid-afternoon	Tea, herbal tea or water Piece of fruit
Tea-time or on arrival at home	Low-fat yoghurt ·
Evening meal	Cheese omelette or scrambled egg with grated cheese, herbs and vegetables

VEGETARIAN MENU 3

Protein packed lunch; carbohydrate evening meal. Ideal on exercise days.

Breakfast	Freshly squeezed orange juice Rehydrated dried prunes or apricots Low-fat yoghurt Coffee, tea or herbal tea (no sugar)
Mid-morning	Tea, herbal tea or water Piece of fruit
Lunch	Pot of low-fat cheese Salad which includes pulses and tomatoes Low-fat yoghurt
Mid-afternoon	Plums, pear, fresh figs or other fruit
Tea-time or on arrival at home	Oatcake or non-sweet biscuit
Evening meal	Pasta with tomato sauce or basil dressing and olive oil Green or mixed salad Bread roll One glass wine (preferably red)

VEGAN MENU 1

Carbohydrate lunch; protein evening meal

Breakfast	Freshly squeezed orange juice
	Rehydrated dried prunes or apricots
	Wholemeal toast with yeast extract spread
	Coffee, tea or herbal tea (no sugar)
Mid-morning	Tea, herbal tea or water
	Pear
Lunch	Couscous with fresh vegetables
	Tea or herbal tea
Mid-afternoon	Fruit
	Tea, herbal tea or water
Tea-time or on arrival at home	Milkshake made with soya milk and banana
Evening meal	Tofu and/or Quorn in sweet and sour sauce made with peppers, tomatoes, onions, spring onions and tinned pineapple chunks (the fruit rules can be relaxed here as cooking tinned pineapple makes it easier to digest)
	Soya sprouts

VEGAN MENU 2

Protein cooked lunch and evening meal. Ideal on busy days when there is little time to prepare food.

Breakfast	Freshly squeezed grapefruit juice
	Porridge made with oats and soya milk
	Coffee, tea or herbal tea (no sugar)
Mid-morning	Tea, herbal tea or water
	Oatcake
Lunch	Vegetable burger, served with vegetables, tomato sauce and soya sprouts
	Tea, herbal tea or water
Mid-afternoon	Pear, peach, plums or other fruit
Tea-time or on arrival at home	One banana
	Tea, herbal tea or water
Evening meal	Tomato or other vegetable soup
	Meal prepared with TVP (frozen or tinned)
	Fresh vegetables
	Tea, herbal tea, water or vegetable juice

VEGAN MENU 3

Carbohydrate lunch; restaurant protein evening meal

Breakfast	Freshly squeezed orange juice
	Porridge made with millet and soya milk
	Coffee, tea or herbal tea (no sugar)
Mid-morning	Fruit or fruit juice
	Tea, herbal tea or water
Lunch	Vegetable soup with bread roll
	Pitta bread with hummus
	Couscous with salad (tabbouleh)
	Bean salad with pasta and tomatoes
Mid-afternoon	Tea, herbal tea, vegetable juice or water
	Fruit
Tea-time or on arrival at home	Oatcake
	Tea, herbal tea or water
Restaurant	Chinese meal with soya and bean curd, soya sprouts, mushrooms (a few cashew nuts in the dish are allowed)

EATING OUT

Sticking to your cellulite-control diet when eating out should not be difficult. Most restaurants offer both protein dishes in the form of meat fish and poultry, and carbohydrate dishes such as pasta, although there is generally a wider choice of protein selections. Beware of fixed menus that offer potatoes or French fries with meat or fish dishes, and ask for extra salad or vegetables instead. Here are some guidelines to help you choose wisely from the menu.

PROTEIN-BASED MEALS

Starters

Choose from:

- Green salad or tomato salad; vegetable soup or thin meat soup; garlic mushrooms; prawns, crab or lobster (no mayonnaise); langoustines; Parma ham; terrine; smoked salmon.
- No bread, rolls or savoury sticks.

Main courses

Choose from:

- Meat, poultry or liver; fish, shellfish, crab or lobster; chilli con carne (no rice).
- All the above should ideally be grilled, roasted, microwaved or poached—or lightly fried if there is no other choice. Accompany them with plenty of vegetables, boiled or steamed, or salad, but no potatoes, rice, pasta, bread or chips.
- A small sliver of cheese but no biscuits.

To drink

- Water; two glasses wine (preferably red) maximum.
- Small coffee to finish, if desired (no sugar).

CARBOHYDRATE-BASED MEALS

Starters

Choose from:

- Green salad or tomato salad; vegetable soup; garlic mushrooms.
- Bread or roll is allowed.

Main courses

Choose from:

- Pasta with vegetable sauce, tomato sauce, basil or herb sauce; couscous with vegetables; rice pilaff with vegetables; noodles with soya sprouts, vegetables, onions, ginger or similar; soya-based meals such as miso or tempeh.
- All can be accompanied with salad or vegetables.

To drink

- Water; two glasses of wine (preferably red) maximum. Small coffee to finish, if desired (no sugar).

ORIENTAL MEALS

Protein-based dishes

Choose:

- Meat, poultry, fish or shellfish, but leave out the rice and noodles. Crispy dishes are very fatty, so avoid these as well.

Carbohydrate-based dishes

Choose:

- Noodles, rice and fermented bean dishes with vegetables, or miso- or tempeh-based dishes, again with rice or noodles.

INDIAN MEALS

Because Indian food can be quite spicy, the temptation is to eat rice, chapatis and other carbohydrates with a main protein meal to balance the spices. Obviously in a food-combining regime this is not ideal. The solution is to eat milder, less spicy protein dishes, without rice. If you like rice, then choose a carbohydrate-based meal such as dahl or lentils so that you can have the spices and the rice. Indian food can be quite fatty, so be very careful in your choice of dishes.

Protein-based dishes

Choose:

- Beef, chicken or shellfish. Kebabs and tandoori dishes contain less fat than the conventional curries. Avoid lamb dishes as these can be quite fatty.
- Bhajis and fried poppadoms are very high in fat and should be avoided.

Carbohydrate-based dishes

Choose:

- Lentil, dahl, bean and pea curries with rice and naan bread if wished.
- Accompany with salad.

GREEK MEALS

Protein-based dishes

Start with:

- A salad of tomatoes, cucumbers, peppers and even a few olives. Shellfish and tuna may also be taken as a starter.
- Avoid taramasalata, hummus, feta and fried vegetables since these are all high in fat.
- For the **main course**, choose meat, fish or shellfish, preferably as kebabs or grilled steaks, or baked in a tomato sauce.
- Accompany with vegetables.
- Greek yoghurt to finish if wished.

Carbohydrate-based dishes

Start with:

- A salad; stuffed tomatoes; stuffed peppers; stuffed vine leaves or potatoes with garlic.

- For the **main course**, choose pasta with tomato sauce, basil and other herbs. Stuffed tomatoes, stuffed peppers and vegetable risotto are also good choices.
- Greek yoghurt to finish if wished.

IF YOU ARE EATING IN A CANTEEN

Many canteens or works' restaurants now include a good range of healthy choices. However, when making protein choices do make sure your meat or fish is not swimming in fat. If there really is no choice between greasy meat, fish in batter, fried egg and cheese dishes, then choose fish in batter and remove the batter, or opt for cold meats if they are available. Eat plenty of vegetables or salad with the meal and finish with a low-fat yoghurt. If you don't like the look of the vegetables, be prepared to take in a few carrots to eat raw.

If you prefer to have a carbohydrate meal, baked potatoes in their jackets are a good choice, as is pasta or couscous with a tomato or vegetable sauce, accompanied with lots of vegetables or salad. Again, if the vegetable choices are poor, then take in your own to eat raw. Finish with a low-fat yoghurt. If you opt for sandwiches, have a salad sandwich, pitta bread with salad or a French roll with salad. Other cold meals could include pasta salad or pasta salad with beans.

Remember, whether opting for a protein or carbohydrate meal, if fruit is on offer, save it for your mid-afternoon snack—not with your meal.

PACKED LUNCH IDEAS

If you don't have a canteen or restaurant at work or you prefer to give it a wide berth, here are some ideas for making your own packed lunches. Do make the effort to prepare something tasty as you'll be less tempted to snack on biscuits and crisps in the afternoon.

Protein-based packed lunches

Choose from the following. Use spices, herbs and garlic to brighten up your lunch.

- Cold meat: chicken, beef, turkey, lamb or pork; cold fish: smoked salmon, tuna or salmon in brine; hard-boiled egg; low-fat cottage cheese.

- Accompany with lots of salad vegetables—lettuce, cucumber, tomatoes, radishes, peppers, carrots and other raw vegetables.
- Finish with a low-fat yoghurt.

Carbohydrate-based packed lunches

Choose from the following. Don't forget the spices, herbs and garlic for that extra kick.

- Bean salad; pasta salad or pasta salad with beans; rice salad with beans; use salad fillings for pitta bread, sandwiches, rolls or French bread.
- Accompany or mix the above with lots of salad vegetables such as lettuce, cucumber, radishes, green and red peppers, tomatoes, carrots and other raw vegetables.
- Finish with a low-fat yoghurt.

THE CELLULITE-CONTROL DIET GUIDELINES

1 Avoid artificial colourings and preservatives.
2 Remove artificial sweeteners from your diet.
3 Control your sodium intake.
4 Use water intelligently.
5 Cut out excess fat.
6 Cut out excess sugar.
7 Limit your intake of alcohol; choose red wine.
8 Limit your intake of coffee.
9 Increase your vegetable and salad intake.
10 Separate fruit from main meals.
11 Separate protein and carbohydrate.

8

TACKLING YOUR DIETARY PROBLEMS

It is essential to tackle any underlying dietary problems if you are to treat cellulite successfully

DEALING WITH FOOD ALLERGIES AND INTOLERANCES

Food allergies and intolerances may cause cellulite and should be investigated

If you suspect that an allergy or intolerance to one or more foods is contributing to your cellulite, you may need to follow an elimination diet to identify the culprit food(s). Blood tests may highlight certain allergies, skin tests others, but there is no single laboratory or clinical investigation other than an elimination diet that can provide an accurate diagnosis of food allergy or intolerance.

However, don't start making radical changes in your diet without considering the consequences. By eliminating some foods you run the risk of becoming deficient in certain nutrients, so think carefully about how you will approach this and which foods you will substitute in their place. An effective elimination diet will take about three to four weeks to complete successfully, so you need to be absolutely certain about your resolve before commencing. Once you have started, you must continue if you are to reap the benefits. If you stop, all will be lost and you will be back to square one.

First, there must be a suspicion that you have a food allergy or intolerance before you set about your elimination diet. Otherwise it might just be a waste of time and set you off on the wrong track. Only about 20 per cent of people with cellulite suffer from a food allergy or intolerance and these people will invariably have other symptoms that may act as pointers to a diagnosis, so it's worth checking these out first by ticking off any symptoms on the list below. Of course, you may still want to follow the diet to be absolutely certain, so by all means go ahead. But don't be surprised if nothing shows up—you may be one of the lucky 80 per cent, but at least then you will know for sure.

CHECKLIST FOR FOOD ALLERGY OR INTOLERANCE

The following are pointers to the suspicion of a food allergy or intolerance

1 Current symptoms

Skin: eczema, urticaria (hives), itches

Ears, nose, throat, eyes: sneezing, wheezing, asthma, persistent cough, catarrh, runny nose, blocked nose, itchy nose, itchy eyes

Joints and muscles: aching joints, arthritis, muscle fatigue, muscle pain

Mouth and digestive system: mouth ulcers, sore tongue, sore throat, indigestion, nausea, vomiting, abdominal pain, bloating, diarrhoea, constipation, colitis, irritable bowel syndrome, food cravings, weight gain, eating certain foods to relieve symptoms

Head, nerves, energy: headache, irritability, fatigue, depression, hyperactivity

Aesthetic/hormonal: water retention, cellulite, weight gain, difficulty in losing weight, weight fluctuations

2 Family history of allergic disease

• Eczema
• Asthma
• Hay fever
• Migraine
• Urticaria (hives)
• Allergy to certain drugs or foods

3 Past history of potential causes

• Early introduction of non-breast milk
• Severe illness
• Hepatitis A
• Glandular fever
• Intestinal infection, inflammation or damage
• Onset of symptoms after an illness or period of stress

If you have *any* of the current symptoms or a family history of allergic disease or a past history of potential causes, then it is likely that you have a food allergy. The next step is to examine your diet pattern.

DIET PATTERN

Below is a list of common allergic foods. Keep a record of everything you eat over a period of four days and see which of the following food groups feature prominently in your diet or which foods you commonly use as a pick-me-up.

Wheat: bread, pasta, noodles, couscous, semolina, biscuits, sauces, pastries, cakes, bran flakes, Shredded Wheat, Weetabix, Frosties or any cereal, crispbreads

Milk: yoghurt, cheese, ice cream, cream, margarine, butter, sauces

Egg: mayonnaise, quiche, some biscuits, cakes, pasta made with egg

Corn: cornflour, corn syrup, corn flakes, polenta, popcorn, corn chips, cornpops, sweetcorn, tacos

Potato: crisps, chips

Tomato: tomato sauce, tomato flavouring, pizza and pasta dishes

Orange: orange juice

Apple: apple juice, natural sweeteners (for example, in soya milk, tinned fruit)

Chocolate: chocolate bars, chocolate drinks, cakes, biscuits

Coffee

Tea

Alcohol

Chicken

Nuts: walnuts, cashew nuts, hazelnuts, peanuts, almonds

Fish

Shellfish

If you highlight a preponderance of one or more of the above foods in your diet, then there's a good chance you may have a food intolerance or allergy. The next step is to embark on an elimination diet.

THE ELIMINATION DIET

An elimination diet must be followed strictly to give a reliable result

The basic principle of any elimination diet is to exclude the most likely suspect foods from your diet. Although it is often possible to make an educated guess as to which ones you are allergic to or intolerant of, the only reliable method of diagnosis is to exclude all potential problem foods for at least five days. These are likely to be the foods you eat most frequently and that you have been eating over a long period of time.

The average daily diet varies from culture to culture. For instance, rice features frequently in the Asian diet, corn in the American diet, so it is important to be aware of your existing diet before you start, otherwise you could spend a week on a diet that is not a true elimination diet and end up none the wiser. If in doubt, seek professional advice.

Five days is the minimum length of time it takes to clear foodstuffs from the intestines and blood system, and in some cases it may take longer. If your intestines are slow to move, for instance if you have constipation, the clearing out process can be helped by taking a single dose of laxative at the start of the diet. For the sake of your health, it is important not to exceed this dose. Alternatively, a single colonic irrigation (described later on page 130) can be used to empty the large bowel of its unwanted contents and speed up the elimination process.

STAGE ONE: STARTING OUT

1 You may eat *only* foods from the "safe foods" list for at least five days. *Choose only the foods that you eat rarely (less than once a week).* As you will be selecting foods that you don't often eat and excluding basic foods such as bread that would normally form part of your everyday diet, I'm afraid the diet may take a little getting used to, but you will have to be firm with yourself. If you break the diet now, you will be back to square one. Eat to satisfy your hunger and forget about the normal food conventions and food-combining principles. If you fancy a lamb chop for breakfast, then have it!

2 You can eat these "safe foods" raw, cooked, roasted, boiled or fried, providing you use only the ingredients allowed. You will have to plan ahead—for instance you may need to prepare a "safe" packed meal to take to work or on any occasion you are going to be away from home.

3 If you are indeed allergic or intolerant, as the days pass you will notice a change in your symptoms in either of the following ways.

You may feel much better—almost straight away. This is more often the case with children, but adults sometimes respond in a similar way.

However, more likely you will feel worse in the beginning. As the foods or food products that are causing an allergic reaction pass out of your system, the body may suffer withdrawal symptoms such as headaches, fatigue, leg pains or general malaise. This is a positive sign that the body is clearing away the allergy. Such symptoms tend to last about two to three days on average, although very allergic people may suffer for a little longer.

4 If the withdrawal symptoms are particularly unpleasant, you may try to relieve them by taking some vitamin C (up to 1g every four hours) or sodium bicarbonate (up to two teaspoons in water every four hours). Vitamin C, if taken in excess, causes diarrhoea; you will soon know if you have taken too much. And remember, diarrhoea reduces the absorption of the contraceptive pill, so you may need to take some extra form of contraception. If necessary, seek your doctor's advice.

5 Normally, the withdrawal symptoms disappear before the fifth day. If they don't, continue the diet for another few days. You need to have at least two days of improvement before starting the second stage of the diet.

SAFE FOODS

Choose only foods from the following list.

Starch: rice, rice flour, rice cakes, yams, buckwheat, sago, eddoes, cassava (manioc, gari).

Meat, poultry, game: lamb, duck, pheasant, quail, venison, ostrich.

Fish: salmon, cod, herring, mackerel, halibut or any fresh or frozen fish but not fish products (for example, fish fingers, fish in batter).

Vegetables: artichoke, asparagus, broccoli, cabbage, cauliflower, celery, Chinese leaf, courgettes, cress, leeks, marrow, parsnip, peas, peppers, runner beans, sprouts, turnip, runner beans.

Pulses: beans, lentils, peas, haricot beans (but not baked beans).

Fruits: blackberries, blueberries, kiwi, melon, passion fruit, pawpaw, pears, pineapple, raspberries, star fruit, strawberries.

Dried fruits: apricots, dates, figs, mangoes, peaches, prunes (all organically dried).

Oil: olive, safflower, sesame, walnut, grapeseed.

Miscellaneous: avocado, olives, honey.

Seasonings: salt, pepper, herbs.

Drinks: mineral water, herbal tea (made with mineral water), pineapple juice, soya milk.

MEAL SUGGESTIONS

As the elimination diet is made up of foods that you probably rarely eat, you may find it monotonous and boring. I'm afraid you will just have to grin and bear it! However, you might like to try some of the combinations below.

Breakfast

- Fresh fruit from list
- Fruit compote made from rehydrated dried fruits and/or fresh fruits from list
- Rice pudding made with rice and soya milk, sweetened with honey
- Rice cakes with avocado

Lunch

- Meat from list, grilled with oil from list (if wished) and herbs
- Vegetables from list, boiled
- Rice, yam or eddoes, boiled
- Fruit salad, using fruits from list

Packed lunch

- Cold meat from list
- Salad ingredients from list
- Olives
- Rice cakes
- Fresh or dried fruits from list

Evening meal

- Avocado salad as starter, using salad ingredients from list
- Meat from list, roasted, microwaved or grilled with oil from list (if wished) and herbs

or

- Fish from list, grilled or microwaved or made into kebabs or baked in paper with herbs and vegetables from list
- Rice cooked in meat stock
- Yam or eddoes, boiled
- Cassava cooked in water or home-made meat stock
- Globe artichoke, boiled then roasted or fried in oil from list

Snacks

- Soya milkshake made from soya milk, fruit from list and honey
- Rice cake and avocado
- Dried fruits from list

Sunday lunch

- Soup made from vegetable or meat stock, thickened with rice flour and flavoured with herbs
- Meat, poultry or game from list, roasted
- Vegetables from list, boiled
- Artichokes, boiled then roasted
- Salad made using ingredients from list, with dressing made from walnut or sesame oil and honey
- Fruit salad or compote made from fresh and/or rehydrated dried fruits from list

STAGE TWO: REINTRODUCTION OF FOODS

By now you should have noticed an improvement in your general health and possibly in the state of your legs. You may have also lost a little weight. Make a note of all these benefits. Now you have to find out exactly which food or foods were causing the problems by reintroducing one food each day. This phase is just as important as stage one and needs to be taken slowly, carefully and thoroughly if you are to benefit fully. You will be looking for a re-occurrence of symptoms as you introduce each food, and also a change in your heart rate, although this second factor may not always be present.

During this stage you can continue eating any foods from the "safe foods" list, but you will need to set aside a certain time each day to test the suspect foods. After eating the food, you will need at least an hour, during which time you will be recording your pulse rate. You should sit quietly during this hour. You may read, write, watch TV or use the computer, but you should not undertake any strenuous activity that will lead to a rise in your pulse rate.

HOW TO PROCEED

1 Set aside a special time for testing the suspect food. The food should be eaten on an empty stomach, and you should not eat any-thing afterwards for a period of three hours, so make sure you eat a

reasonably large quantity. If you are out all day, it is best to eat "safe" foods during the day and then to test foods on your return. If you are at home all day you can test foods at any time that suits you.

2 Prepare the food if necessary, choosing from the above "safe foods" list. Before eating the food, sit quietly and take your radial pulse. This can be found by pressing gently with your middle and index finger on the inner surface of the other wrist, about two centimetres down from the crease between your hand and your wrist, just to the outer side of the tendon. Count the number of pulsations over sixty seconds. This will give you your resting pulse rate. You may find it easier to use an analogue watch with a second hand rather than a digital watch. Make a note of this pulse.

3 Eat the food. Set a timer or record the time.

4 After eating the food, record your pulse at ten-minute intervals over a period of one hour. Make a note of each reading.

5 During this hour, make a note of any symptoms that occur, however bizarre they may seem at the time. The aim is to see if a pattern arises as the testing continues.

6 Wait a good three hours before eating anything else. Make sure you only eat foods from the "safe" list. Record any further symptoms that may develop, even after the first hour has passed.

7 The next day, proceed in the same way to test another food.

8 Usually, any adverse reaction generated by testing a food will have subsided by the following day. However, if you did your testing very late in the day or tested meat, the symptoms may hang around until the following morning. Eat only "safe" foods until the symptoms have subsided. A prolonged reaction should normally last no longer than twenty-four hours.

9 After one week, look at your results. You will be able to identify which foods you can eat safely and which cause an adverse reaction. An allergic or intolerant reaction will manifest itself in one of the following ways:

- The re-occurrence of symptoms already familiar to you (bloating, headaches, etc).
- An increase in your resting pulse rate by ten beats a minute.
- An increase in weight the next day.
- A deterioration in the state of your legs (water retention, worsening of cellulite or a feeling of heaviness).

The culprit foods should be classed as "allergic" and should be avoided from now on. Any foods that have been tested with no adverse reactions can be added to the "safe" list. This will increase the choice of foods available to you, and it is very important to eat as varied a diet as possible for optimum health.

10 Continue testing foods for the next week or so until you have tested all the foods. You will end up with a list of "safe" foods, a list of culprit foods and perhaps a few "don't knows." Test these "don't knows" again, but always leave a gap of five days before retesting the same food, or foods in the same group (for example, milk and yoghurt).

FOODS TO BE REINTRODUCED

You can also add other foods that you eat frequently to this list. As a guide, this is a list of the most frequently eaten (and thus trigger) foods that need to be tested individually in the reintroduction stage. They are given here in alphabetical order, but you may test them in a sequence that fits into your daily routine. Remember that you are testing a single food at a time, so foods that frequently contain or are taken with others eg. chocolate, omelette and coffee, must be tested in their pure form. It is recommended that you try a few "useful" foods such as meats, fruit and starches in the first week so that you can identify your safe foods and make up a balanced diet as soon as possible. The next week try a few more staples, and only when you have plenty of basic foods in your diet should you start to introduce things like alcohol, chocolate, tea and coffee.

Here's the list of foods to be reintroduced:

Alcohol
Apples: fresh apples
Bananas: fresh bananas, uncooked
Beef: grilled or roast
Carrots: fresh carrots only, eaten raw
Cheese: Cheddar cheese only
Chicken: grilled or roasted
Chocolate: plain chocolate only
Coffee: drunk black. (NB: Coffee increases the pulse rate, so when testing coffee there is no need to take your pulse. Just check for any symptoms.)
Corn: corn on the cob, popcorn, corn chips
Eggs: boiled, scrambled, fried with grapeseed oil or made into omelette (no milk)
*Fish: fresh fish, grilled, microwaved or poached (include only if fish not eaten on elimination diet)
Lemons: fresh lemons only

Milk: fresh milk, whole, skimmed or semi-skimmed
*Nuts: peanuts, almonds, walnuts, cashew nuts
Oranges: fresh oranges only
Pork: grilled or roasted
Potatoes: boiled, mashed or microwaved
Rice: only include if not eaten on elimination diet
*Shellfish: raw or cooked
Tea: drunk black. (NB: Tea raises the pulse rate, so when testing tea, there is no need to take your pulse. Just check for any symptoms.)
Tomatoes: fresh tomatoes only
Wheat: pasta, water biscuits only
Yeast tablets: take three in water (to test sensitivity to yeast in bread, buns, Danish Pastries etc.)

NB: Cheese, chocolate and nuts are included here for the allergy diagnosis diet. Remember that these contain too much fat and/or sugar to be included in the cellulite control diet.

*Nuts, fish and shellfish can be harmful in certain allergic individuals. If you know or suspect that you are allergic to these, or other foodstuffs, check with your doctor before testing these foods.

WHAT TO DO NEXT

What you now need to do is to devise a nutritionally balanced diet based on "safe" foods. If you are allergic to just one or two items, as is usually the case, this should not be a problem. Remember that if you are allergic to a certain food, you will be allergic to that food in all its forms. So, an allergy to milk means that you will also be allergic to yoghurt, cheese, milk powder, whey, bread, cakes or biscuits containing milk, milk chocolate and so on.

With some vegetables and fruits, particularly carrots, apples, peaches, pears and tomatoes, the allergic symptoms are lessened if the food is cooked, as the heat destroys some of their "allergic" potential. If you suffer an allergic reaction to a raw item you may wish to try cooking the vegetable or fruit and see if you suffer in the same way. The only food where the allergic reaction is heightened after cooking is milk. Dried milk, sterilised milk and milk puddings cause more reaction than their raw base.

If you are allergic to several foods, you may need help from your doctor or nutritionist to work out a healthy diet. You do not want to replace a balanced diet, albeit one that includes foods to which you are allergic, with an allergy-free but nutritionally deficient diet. You may also need to consult a doctor who is trained in dealing with complex food allergies.

WILL I BE ALLERGIC TO THAT FOOD FOR EVER?

Although some allergies may remain with you for life, most diminish once the problem food is removed from the diet. After you have avoided the culprit food for six months, you may try eating it again. There is a good chance that you will not suffer any symptoms, in which case the food can be reintroduced occasionally into your diet. However, don't fall into the trap of eating that food too often again, otherwise you run the risk of a re-occurrence of symptoms.

- Food allergies can cause cellulite and need to be investigated.
- To highlight the culprit foods, a strict elimination diet should be necessary, followed by a gradual reintroduction of foods.

DEALING WITH SUGAR CRAVINGS AND HYPOGLYCAEMIA

Replace simple sugars with complex carbohydrates

Your intake of simple sugars such as those found in chocolate, biscuits, dried fruits and cakes should be reduced to a minimum in a cellulite-control diet. That's all very well, but what happens if you suffer an insurmountable craving for sugar, together with all the tell-tale signs of irritability, poor concentration, hunger, mood swings and light-headedness?

Hypoglycaemia, or low blood sugar, can present itself as any or all of these symptoms and defy diagnosis for some time. During this time, the sufferer consumes more sugar in the misguided belief that this will help. This relieves the symptoms in the short term by causing the blood sugar level to rise temporarily, only to plummet again soon afterwards, leading to a vicious circle. More sugar, more insulin, fewer trace elements. More hypoglycaemic attacks. And more fat storage.

This vicious cycle must be interrupted if you are to rectify the situation, and this can be done relatively easily. All it takes is a little motivation. What you need to do is to ban all simple sugars from your diet to avoid fluctuations in the blood sugar level and increase your intake of complex carbohydrates such as rice, pasta, beans, pulses, millet and buckwheat. These complex carbohydrates will slowly release their sugar content and help maintain a stable blood sugar level. In this instance, potatoes and bread are considered as simple sugars and should be avoided, since they are easily digested and their sugar is rapidly released.

This means having some form of complex carbohydrate for breakfast, lunch and with the evening meal. Your food-combining regime will have to go out of the window for a while, unless you are able to live on pulses, but once your blood sugar level is more stable again, you can skip the carbohydrate with the evening meal.

VITAMIN AND MINERAL SUPPLEMENTS FOR SUGAR CRAVING

Increasing your intake of complex carbohydrates may cure your sugar craving, but more often than not a little extra help is required. A high sugar intake can reduce the amount of the trace elements chromium, zinc, nickel and cobalt in the body. Without these, the insulin secretion process loses its fine tuning, which results in swings in sugar levels. Supplementing your diet with these trace elements will help keep the blood sugar level stable.

Chromium

Chromium can become deficient in those people who have repeatedly consumed a high-sugar diet and who have used up their body stores of chromium by continually secreting insulin. The symptoms of chromium deficiency are exactly the same as the symptoms of sugar craving: hunger, weakness, light-headedness, desire for sugars and sweet things. Chromium is now available in an organic (and therefore easily absorbed) form, commonly known as glucose tolerance factor, and this can be obtained from most chemists and health food stores. A regular dose of 100mcg per day will improve glucose tolerance, reduce sugar craving and remove hypoglycaemic attacks.

Chromium is also available in combination with other vitamins and minerals. This latter formulation may be more useful, as single deficiencies are rare. It is quite likely that whatever has caused the hypoglycaemia has also caused other deficiencies.

Zinc-nickel-cobalt oligosol

Oligotherapy is a French speciality which uses tiny amounts of trace minerals to treat various disorders. Sugar craving, weakness and hunger can be treated by a zinc-nickel-cobalt solution which should be taken in minute doses just under the tongue, guaranteeing good absorption. Two to three ampoules taken each day for twenty-one days is normally sufficient to rectify the problem. Not only will this help reduce sugar cravings but it can also have a beneficial effect on weight loss. A controlled trial showed that a zinc-nickel-cobalt solution taken in conjunction with a weight-reducing diet can aid weight loss by an extra 2 or 3kg over a six-week period.

Vitamins B1, B2, B6, magnesium, chromium, zinc

Pre-menstrual sugar cravings respond well to supplementation with vitamins B1, B2 and B6, magnesium, chromium and zinc. These are often available in combination with other vitamins and can also help other pre-menstrual symptoms such as fatigue, mood swings, irritability and poor concentration. In addition, there is now a good selection of well-balanced supplements suitable for women of reproductive age and those who are nearing the menopause, available from reputable vitamin suppliers. Never exceed the manufacturer's recommended dosage and, if in doubt, consult your doctor or nutritionist.

• Hypoglycaemia responds well to dietary treatments and supplements.

DEALING WITH ABDOMINAL BLOATING, DIGESTIVE PROBLEMS AND CONSTIPATION

Bloating, digestive problems and constipation have many causes and must be treated in order to deal effectively with cellulite

ABDOMINAL BLOATING

Abdominal bloating is uncomfortable, unpleasant, unsightly and disturbs the normal posture by pushing out the abdomen and tilting back the pelvis. A bloated abdomen does not allow the normal thoraco-abdominal pump to function quite so effectively and thus prevents the normal return of lymph. There are several approaches to the treatment of bloating, depending on the underlying problem.

Lactobacillus (acidophilus or bifido bacteria)

Lactobacillus is one of many friendly bowel flora or bacteria that live in our intestines. Normally, these friendly bacteria aid digestion, produce B-complex vitamins and fend off more toxic bacteria. However, the normal bowel flora is fairly fragile and is easily destroyed by repeated administration of antibiotics and/or a diet rich in sugars and refined carbohydrates. In some instances, the normal flora can be replaced by a less friendly flora, more akin to yeasts and fungi, that ferment and produce gas, using up essential vitamins and minerals in the process. This causes bloating and wind as well as symptoms such as sugar cravings, mood swings, fatigue and recurrent vaginal thrush. These symptoms, often known as candidiasis, are common in those people who have managed to upset their normal bowel flora and allowed yeasts and fungi to replace them.

To rectify this, a bowel flora replacement supplement such as lactobacillus can be taken to re-establish a more normal bowel flora. Make sure the supplement has been prepared in an acid-resistant form so that it can survive the effects of the acid in the stomach. Lactobacillus supplementation should always be taken in conjunction with a diet that is low in sugar and high in protein, vegetables and complex carbohydrates such as beans and pulses to minimise the overgrowth of yeast. Foods similar to yeasts should also be avoided as these can mimic the effects of yeast in the intestines. In addition, a vitamin and mineral supplement should always be taken because the abnormal floras rapidly deplete the body's stores of essential vitamins and minerals. Vitamins B1, B2, B6, C and E, zinc and magnesium are the most commonly deficient vitamins and these may be taken separately or in specially formulated combinations.

Some yoghurts contain lactobacillus and these are useful for those people who do not necessarily need or want to take bowel flora replacement supplements. Make sure that the yoghurt stipulates "bifido," "lactobacillus" or "acidophilus" on the pot. "Live" yoghurt is not enough. One or two pots of bifido-rich yoghurt a day will maintain a good bowel flora. Onions, leeks and carrots are also excellent foodstuffs for stimulating a healthy bowel flora.

Poor digestion of cellulose

If abnormal bowel floras are not the cause of the abdominal bloating, then it is necessary to look further for a possible culprit. Certain foods such as beans, baked beans, broccoli, chickpeas, cabbage, bran, peanuts, brussels sprouts and onions are commonly known to cause bloating and wind in some people. All these foods contain complex carbohydrates known as celluloses which are sometimes unable to be digested by our natural digestive system and this is what causes the bloating and wind. Some people may steer clear of these foods to avoid these symptoms, yet by doing so, they can be denying themselves healthy anti-cellulite foods.

There are a number of products on the market that can help aid digestion of these foods, or at least limit the effects of the gas produced during their digestion; Galactozyme and peppermint oil are the most effective.

Galactozyme: This is a new supplement that digests the hitherto indigestible cellulose and therefore prevents bloating. Two tablets taken with the very first mouthful of the problem food is sufficient to prevent bloating. If the bloating is particularly troublesome, galactozyme can be taken before every meal that contains vegetables.

Peppermint oil: Peppermint oil also helps relieve bloating and cramps by reducing the effect of air on the intestines. Peppermints can help, but peppermint oil is the active ingredient. This can be prepared in an enteric coating, so that the capsule survives the stomach acid and only opens up in the intestine. Thus the peppermint oil is released exactly where it is needed, in the intestines.

CONSTIPATION

Constipation itself can cause bloating and can also impair the lymphatic drainage of the legs. Although there are many causes of constipation, there are a number of natural remedies that can help cure it. If, after trying these, the constipation is no better, then you should seek your doctor"s advice.

The bowel is at its most active in the morning, so this is the best time to aim to increase its function. There are various ways of doing this.

Water and magnesium

Drink three glasses of warm mineral water, preferably one that is high in magnesium (for example, Vittel), before breakfast. Magnesium is a natural laxative and is available as Epsom salts from pharmacies. If you cannot obtain high magnesium water and you need a little help with constipation, then add two flat teaspoons to a litre of water.

Time and relaxation

Always give yourself time to go to the toilet, never hurry. Relax. Get up ten minutes earlier in the morning if necessary so that you're not rushed. Never put off the desire to open your bowels, where possible. It's a bad habit to get into, and eventually the bowels will no longer send out or respond to the "I'm full" message.

Activity

Aim to increase your exercise and activity during the day. Even if your job is sedentary, get off your chair or get out of the car and do a few stretching exercises. Not only will this help your bowels, but it will also help your legs.

Fibre

Make sure your diet is high in fibre. Foods such as vegetables, wholemeal cereals, bran, beans and pulses are all high in fibre. Always remember to drink enough water to allow the fibre to expand fully and do its job. Some fibres, such as bran, can cause abdominal cramps. If this is the case, switch to a more gentle form of fibre such as vegetables, oats, beans and pulses. If this is to no avail, then try fibre supplements available in health food shops or from your GP.

High-fibre foods: All Bran; dried rehydrated apricots; dried reconstituted figs; dried rehydrated prunes; blackcurrants; Weetabix; cornflakes; rye crispbread; wholemeal bread; Ready Brek; green peas; lentils; beans such as haricot beans; baked beans; cabbage, artichoke; spinach.
    Fibre supplements: kelp; linseed; Fybogel; Isogel; oat bran; rice bran; wheat bran.

Food allergies

Check that you do not have any food allergies (see earlier in this chapter). Quite often, an allergy to a certain food can cause constipation, and food allergies are often associated with other symptoms.

Disturbed bowel flora

Think about the possibility of a bowel flora disturbance, especially if you have been taking antibiotics or have had a high-sugar diet for some time. Treat with lactobacillus (in yoghurt or supplement form) and ensure you follow a low-sugar, high-protein diet. If you do not see any improvement, then consult your doctor.

Colonic irrigation

Colonic irrigation involves the gentle removal of large bowel contents using a water-based enema. Water is introduced via a tube fed through the anus and washes out the faecal contents. Colonic irrigation does benefit those who are chronically constipated or who have digestive problems. There is no doubt that faeces in the large bowel that should be long gone cause all sorts of toxic problems and affect your health and wellbeing. Colonic irrigation is not a do-it-yourself technique, you need to be treated by a skilled therapist. Private clinics and health centres often have a colonic therapist who should be trained in the procedure.

In terms of an anti-cellulite regime, colonic irrigation is useful for those people with chronic, longstanding constipation and for people who are just about to embark on a food elimination diet. However, it is no substitute for a good diet, attention to the bowel flora and good bowel habits.

- Abdominal bloating, digestive problems and constipation require treatment and can be overcome by altering your diet or by taking supplements.

PROTECTING YOURSELF AGAINST FREE RADICAL DAMAGE

Some people may need to supplement their diet with antioxidant vitamins and minerals

Beta-carotene, vitamin C, vitamin E, manganese and selenium are antioxidant vitamins and minerals which protect the small blood vessels against the damaging effects of free radicals from smoking, chemicals, sunlight and pollution. Fresh fruit and vegetables, particularly the brightly coloured ones, are the best dietary source of antioxidants, so aim to include plenty of these in your diet. Some individuals who are sensitive to certain chemicals and foods are less likely to be able to detoxify free radicals because of a deficiency in their neutralising enzyme system and therefore need to supplement their diet with antioxidant vitamins and minerals.

Like insulin, enzymes have helpers in the form of trace minerals and vitamins that help them function to their highest capacity. By supplementing these enzyme helpers, the effects of the free radicals can be limited. There are many suitable vitamin and mineral supplements available. Some vitamins work as free-radical scavengers in their own right.

- There are some individuals who are sensitive to certain chemicals and foods such as make-ups, creams, alcohol, cigarette smoke. It seems that these people are less able to detoxify free radicals because of a deficiency in their neutralising enzyme system. If you are sensitive to chemicals and/or foods, consider supplementing your diet with anti-oxidant vitamins and minerals.

9

ESSENTIAL EXERCISE

A good exercise routine is fundamental to any cellulite treatment regime

There are many ways that exercise can help both in the treatment and prevention of cellulite and it should therefore form an integral part of any anti-cellulite routine. Exercise improves the circulation and lymphatic and venous drainage, and aids the removal of fat.

However, before rushing into a new exercise regime, you should consider carefully what other complementary steps need to be taken. You will need additional help to encourage the removal of fat by the use of creams, aromatherapy or professional treatment. Remember that fat is preferentially released from the upper body and stored on the lower body, so the last thing you want is for any fat removed by your anti-cellulite efforts to be redeposited on your thighs. Exercise will help burn up the fat before it has a chance to do so.

Regular exercise, at least three times a week for a minimum of twenty minutes, will also increase your basal metabolic rate and help you burn more calories, not just while you are exercising but also afterwards. If you are on a weight-loss diet, exercise will help ensure you don't lose muscle mass.

A natural by-product of exercise is lactic acid. Lactic acid, like vitamin C, is a natural chelator; in other words, it clears away any free radicals, cholesterol and other debris that would otherwise collect inside the blood vessels. This debris is known as plaque. It's like descaling a kettle or defurring a pipe. If this debris were not removed, it would encourage the formation of plaques which would eventually block the blood vessels, particularly the small ones. Once it has done its job, the lactic acid needs to be cleared from the tissues, and a good cool-down and stretch session at the end of your exercise period will help speed this process along.

Any exercise that involves the legs, such as walking, cycling, dancing and trampolining, causes the muscles of the calves and thighs to contract. The contraction of these leg muscles exerts a pumping action on the otherwise sluggish veins and lymphatics, and pumps venous blood and lymph fluid back up towards the heart. Regular flexing, stretching and extending the foot as in dancing, particularly ballroom dancing, improves the return of lymph to the heart by stimulating the plantar return reflex.

Specific abdominal exercises will tone and strengthen the abdomen, and strong abdominal muscles improve the functioning of the thoraco-abdominal pump which returns venous blood and lymph to the heart. Strengthening the abdominal muscles will benefit posture and have the effect of pulling the pelvis back into alignment and freeing a tight inguinal canal (the narrow channel in the groin) in cases of bad posture and lordosis. The resulting release of tension in the inguinal canal allows the unrestricted return of lymph and venous blood.

Exercise is a natural anti-depressant and helps combat the effects of stress and pressure in our everyday lives. Regular exercise allows the brain to release morphine-like, naturally occurring endorphins into the bloodstream which can enhance our mood and protect us from the harmful effects of stress. Our sense of wellbeing increases and we feel more at ease with ourselves. This relaxed state enables the body to "unblock" its own self-healing channels, thus allowing us to benefit more greatly from any treatment procedure that we may follow.

- Regular exercise increases the rate at which we burn calories.
- Exercise produces lactic acid which cleanses the arteries, thereby improving blood supply.
- Exercising the legs encourages the return of venous blood and lymph to the heart.
- Movements that stretch and flex the feet encourage the return of lymph.
- Strong abdominal muscles allow the thoraco-abdominal pump to function well and return venous blood and lymph to the circulation.
- Abdominal exercises encourage good posture.
- Regular exercise acts as a natural anti-depressant, combats stress and increases our sense of wellbeing.

EXERCISE FOR DYSMORPHISM

Dysmorphism sufferers need to exercise both the upper and lower body

Remember that dysmorphism tends to affect people who overwork the legs without paying attention to the upper torso. Footballers are typical sufferers, but women who concentrate on exercising the legs at the expense of the upper body can also be affected. Sufferers are aware of their disposition to "big thighs" but do not realise that it is a real medical condition that can be treated. Many therapists simply advise such people not to exercise. Although this may help the problem in the short term, it is certainly not a long-term solution since exercise is important not just for the treatment of cellulite but also for general health. What is needed is a properly tailored exercise routine in conjunction with appropriate treatment for the circulation, veins and lymphatic drainage in order to cure dysmorphism.

Any exercise regime must ensure that both the upper and lower torso are worked equally, although not necessarily at the same time. So, running could be combined with some light weights work on the arms, or cycling combined with badminton or swimming. Stretching is beneficial, as is dancing, running and aqua aerobics. Avoid exercise that overuses the front thigh muscles (quadriceps), for instance kickboxing or high-impact aerobics, and any leg exercises which involve short, repetitive movements that place the legs under strain and encourage the development of bulk. Instead, choose exercise that takes the legs through a mid or full range of movement.

- Dysmorphism sufferers need to follow a balanced exercise routine that pays attention to both the upper and lower torso.
- Exercise that involves excessive use of the quadriceps should be avoided.
- Exercise that involves short, repetitive movements of the legs is also to be avoided.

MUSCLE – TO BUILD OR NOT TO BUILD

Some women have a greater tendency to gain muscle bulk than others

Why is it that some women seem to build muscle on their legs almost too easily, while others work out regularly in the gym and acquire sleek, toned bodies without acquiring extra unsightly muscle bulk?

Generally, there are two factors that lead to the acquisition of muscle mass. First, it requires the presence of the male hormone testosterone, which is why men build muscle easily. Women, on the other hand, only have small amounts of this hormone in their bodies and therefore its effect is negligible. This is why women will not acquire the kind of muscles we associate with bodybuilders unless they were to follow an extremely intensive regime, usually requiring endless hours of training in the gym and a specialised diet.

The second, more relevant factor relates to basic body shape. Tall, slim individuals with long legs will rarely build muscle mass however much they exercise, even if they work out with weights. The reason for this is that each end of a particular muscle is attached to a bone. If the muscle attachments are far apart, then when that muscle is exercised, it will not develop any substantial mass. Conversely, in a squat individual with short legs, the muscle attachments are much closer together and, thus, the muscle rapidly develops bulk when exercised. So, a relatively short woman with a chunky build is much more likely to build muscle mass than a woman with a tall, slender physique.

Look at weightlifters and long-distance runners. Weight-lifters need a hugely powerful muscle mass to lift a large weight in a short burst of energy, and such people are inevitably short, squat and muscly. Long-distance runners on the other hand need only to carry their own bodyweight, but they need stamina, finely toned muscles and a streamlined shape for speed. That's why they are long, lean and thin.

There's not much you can do to alter your basic body shape, but once you are aware of this connection then at least you can choose the best type of exercise for you. If you are relatively tall and slim, then you can choose almost any exercise you like without fear of building bulk. Also, if you know from past experience that you are a unlikely to build bulk, then go ahead and exercise as you wish.

If, however, you are on the short, squat, even chunky side, or know that you have a tendency to gain bulk, be careful and avoid the type of exercise that involves repetitive movements of the legs, and certainly do not use weights on your legs. Instead, choose exercises that lengthen and stretch the muscle, such as ballroom dancing, swimming, walking (striding) and hill walking.

- Tall, slim women rarely build muscle bulk and may engage in almost any form of exercise.
- Short, squat women may have a tendency to acquire some muscle bulk and need to avoid specific muscle-building exercises for the legs.

HOW MUCH EXERCISE DO I NEED?

Any exercise is better than none

We need about twenty minutes of aerobic exercise three times a week if we are to improve the strength of our heart, lungs and blood vessels and effectively burn fat. Aerobic exercise is any exercise that causes your heart to beat faster and that makes you slightly breathless for the full twenty minutes; for example, brisk walking, running. Ideally, we should start with a brief warm-up and stretch routine, do our twenty minutes of exercise, then cool off and stretch once again.

If you are new to exercising, this might seem a tall order. What I suggest, therefore, is that you start off by doing just as much as you can manage. Start with perhaps just one session a week and build up from there. Always set yourself manageable targets. If you attempt to do too much too soon, you are likely to end up with aches and pains and possibly injure yourself. This will only deter you from continuing and you'll just be giving yourself more stress.

The other way is to get as much exercise as possible during the normal course of the day. Take the stairs instead of the lift; walk to work instead of taking the bus or the car, and walk briskly instead of ambling. Ideally, combine "formal" exercise with an active lifestyle.

Some of the best exercises for an anti-cellulite regime are brisk walking, jogging, trampolining, aqua aerobics, swimming, cycling, step aerobics, dancing and working out with light weights. If you can, choose a form of exercise that will also work your upper body and arms. You may also like to do some additional toning exercise to improve the shape of your legs and undertake some abdominal work to strengthen your tummy muscles and improve your posture (see pages 144–164 for toning exercises).

You might consider joining an exercise class or going along to a gym. Attending a structured exercise class will encourage you to be consistent and therefore obtain better results. It's not always easy to exercise at home unless you are really motivated.

If you have to exercise at home, then you need lots of self-discipline. Set aside a specific period of time for your exercise—the same time each day if possible so that you are more likely to do it. Take the phone off the hook or put the answerphone on to ensure that you are not interrupted. Choose a time when the children are at school or otherwise occupied, and give yourself a good workout. You'll feel great afterwards!

- Although three sessions of exercise per week are recommended, any exercise at all will help your cellulite.
- Unless you are very motivated and can easily work out at home, attending a class will ensure a more rigorous and consistent workout and lead to better results.

WHAT TO WEAR

Choose the best clothing to protect fragile, floppy legs

Heavy legs, loose, floppy cellulite-ridden and waterlogged tissues demand a little more care during exercise than firm cellulite tissue. Legs with cellulite are already suffering from a poor lymphatic drainage, and allowing such tissue to wobble about merely creates more damage to the lymphatics and ultimately makes the cellulite worse. The loose tissue becomes looser, your morale drops—and your new-found exercise regime goes out of the window!

Wearing well-fitting, but not too tight, lycra leggings or support tights gives the underlying lymph vessels the respect they need. If the legs are really heavy, avoid exercise that allows them to wobble about uncontrollably. So, instead of tennis, running and aerobics, choose swimming, cycling, dance, walking or use a step machine, at least until your legs firm up enough to allow you to return to your favourite sport.

- Protect heavy or floppy legs from excessive wobbling during exercise by wearing well-fitting leggings or support tights.

GOOD POSTURE

A good posture will improve your looks and wellbeing as well as help treat cellulite

Good posture is synonymous with good health. The muscles of the back, neck, tummy, shoulders and thighs all contribute to our maintaining a good posture. Unfortunately, because many of us spend a lot of time slouched in a chair, in front of the TV or behind the wheel of a car, the muscles that we use to hold ourselves upright have become lazy, and our bodies suffer as a result. The head tips forwards, the shoulders become rounded, the back slumps and the tummy sticks out. Not only does this look unattractive, it also impairs the way that the body functions. Over a period of time, the body becomes accustomed to this poor posture, but the neck, head and low back complain as the spine adapts to this unnatural position. The inevitable aches and pains that follow affect the quality of our lives, prevent us following a good exercise routine and add to our stress levels.

As poor posture allows the tummy muscles to sag, the pelvis tips forwards and the inguinal canal becomes squashed. Consequently, the normal return of venous blood and lymph is prevented and fluid collects in the tissues of the legs. Strong abdominal muscles, on the other hand, ensure that the pelvis is correctly aligned, taking the pressure off the inguinal canal so that the flow of fluid leaving the legs via the lymph vessels and veins is unimpeded. Strong abdominal muscles also provide the necessary resistance to allow the thoraco-abdominal pump to work at

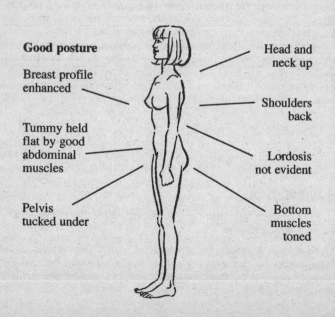

Good posture

Breast profile
enhanced

Tummy held
flat by good
abdominal
muscles

Pelvis
tucked under

Head and
neck up

Shoulders
back

Lordosis
not evident

Bottom
muscles
toned

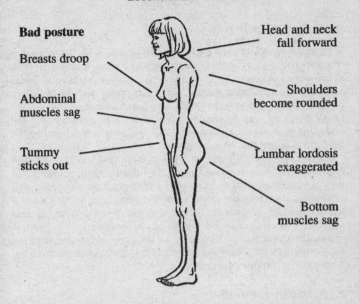

Bad posture

Head and neck
fall forward

Breasts droop

Shoulders
become rounded

Abdominal
muscles sag

Tummy
sticks out

Lumbar lordosis
exaggerated

Bottom
muscles sag

its optimum level and enable the return of venous blood and lymph to the general circulation.

The abdominal muscles work in conjunction with the muscles of the back. If the abdominal muscles are weak, this puts extra stress on the back, and therefore takes up energy. Good posture creating a body that is at ease with itself, will conserve energy and therefore improve energy levels.

It's not always easy to check your own posture. Spend a bit more time in front of the full-length mirror in your underclothes and look critically at your posture. Could you stand a bit taller? Will your tummy tuck in a bit, and your bottom under? Tighten up the tummy muscles. And what about those shoulders? Keep them back. Head up—stand proud. When you are sitting, don't let the head and shoulders droop forward, and keep the tummy muscles tight. You'll be surprise how much better you feel and look. The abdominal exercises on pages 155–158 will go a long way to help improving your posture, but you may feel you need additional help. There are a number of specific techniques such as osteopathy or chiropractic, Alexander technique and Pilates which can all help correct postural problems.

OSTEOPATHY AND CHIROPRACTIC

We tend to associate osteopathy or chiropractic with the treatment of back problems. However, an osteopath or chiropractor will look at the whole structure of the body—the bones, muscles and joints and their intricate relationship. Very often, poor posture results in back and neck pain as some joints stiffen and some muscles tighten to adjust to the misalignment of the body. It is essential that the underlying pain, stiffness and muscle spasm is treated before the postural problem can be rectified.

An osteopath or chiropractor will therefore first use manipulation to ensure that your back and neck are fully in alignment and that your posture is as good as it can be. Then, if necessary, he or she will recommend some exercises to strengthen the tummy muscles and realign the pelvis. In turn, these will aid lymphatic return and improve your chances of getting rid of your cellulite.

Manipulation may be useful on its own or used in combination with other postural, exercise or relaxation techniques such as the Alexander technique or Pilates.

ALEXANDER TECHNIQUE

The Alexander technique is a well-established technique that trains you to be aware of and maintain a balanced posture. Alexander therapists will analyse your posture and aim to rectify it through a series of exercises and postural techniques.

PILATES

The Pilates method looks at the balance between the muscle groups in the whole body. All muscle groups work in pairs, and if one muscle group is weak, this creates an imbalance which places abnormal stress upon the body. Pilates practitioners will therefore assess the function and strength of all the muscles and analyse the effect of any weaknesses. A series of specific, non-muscle bulking exercises will then be recommended to correct any muscle imbalance. Such exercises will be non-weight bearing and will use elastic bands, pulleys and pillows to target specific muscle groups. Special attention is paid to technique. Mirrors are used to help you check your position and ensure the best results. Classes tend to be very small, so that the practitioner can devote sufficient time to each client. After the initial assessment session, classes last between sixty and ninety minutes. At least ten sessions are recommended, although many people find the whole experience so beneficial that they choose to take more.

One particular benefit of the Pilates system as far as cellulite is concerned is that the inner thigh muscles can be strengthened almost exclusively without building muscle on the outer thighs. The inner thigh muscles get very little use in everyday activities and are therefore naturally weak. Consequently, the inner thigh area is a common problem zone, and Pilates offers a direct solution to this problem.

Pilates can also be used to strengthen weak tummy muscles and leg muscles without placing undue strain on weak or tender joints. This is particularly beneficial for those people who have not exercised for some time or who suffer from joint or back pain.

By gently exercising—but never stressing—the muscles, any neck or back pain caused by unequal tension in the muscles can be relieved after just one session. Pilates is excellent for combating stress and muscular tension, and any method that combats stress has to be advantageous in the treatment of cellulite.

- Good posture can improve your looks and your wellbeing.
- Poor posture results in muscular pain and stress and can contribute to cellulite.
- Osteopathy/chiropractic, Alexander technique and Pilates can improve posture and help relieve muscle tension and stress.

ELIMINATE STRESS

Stress can play a key role in the development of cellulite

Adrenaline released under conditions of stress can cause cellulite or make existing cellulite worse by promoting the storage of fat. Stress can encourage the development of cellulite on the legs, but mostly it tends to occur on the tummy, just beneath the ribs or on the back of the neck. In many cases, it's simply not possible, or indeed desirable, to completely remove stress from our lives. What we can do, however, is to boost our defences against stress and help protect our bodies from its more damaging effects.

Recent research has shown that any health problem that lasts more than six months sets up its own perpetuating short-circuit in the brain. Let's divert a little bit and talk about back pain as an example to explain this. Lifting a heavy weight may cause a back pain—torn ligaments, bruised muscles and perhaps a pinched nerve. Ouch!! Agony!! After a few days of rest, however, the pain subsides. No more pain. End of story. Supposing, however, that the pain does not go away, for whatever reason. Simple movements such as lifting, driving, etc. now cause the symptoms to reappear as they put a strain on the back. Ouch again!! Note here that at the moment the pain is still caused by events related to the back.

After a long time, however, it's not only physical factors that influence the pain. Psychological ones, such as fatigue, cold weather, depression, stress, do as well. The illness-perpetuating short-circuit has been set up. So not only does the individual have to alter his way of life, he has to find ways of overcoming stress, improving his outlook and generally making himself more resistant to those outside influences. It's the same with cellulite. Once cellulite has taken hold and established itself as a familiar feature of the body, in order to get rid of cellulite we also have to get rid of any accompanying stress as well as the underlying cause.

Exercise, along with techniques such as yoga, Alexander technique, Pilates, head and neck massage, cranial osteopathy (a massage and manipulation technique to the head and neck) and aromatherapy, can aid relaxation, and help us to cope with and minimise the effects of stress. In some instances, particularly when stress is a cause or a predominant feature of the cellulite problem, then a good relaxation programme, followed correctly, can be just as effective as exercise in helping to reduce cellulite.

If you just don't seem to find the time to relax, you may need extra incentive and help. The appropriate practitioner can show you the best techniques, and these will help you control and, indeed, shift cellulite more effectively. Of course, exercise is still important, and you will still need to think of ways of increasing your activity levels in everyday life, even if you choose not to follow a "formal" exercise plan.

- Stress can cause cellulite or make existing cellulite worse.
- Stress must be effectively treated if the cellulite is to be shifted.
- Choose a method of relaxation that suits you.

EFFECTIVE EXERCISES FOR AN ANTI-CELLULITE REGIME

The following exercises should be used in conjunction with your regular exercise routine, be it walking, step aerobics or dancing, and will help tone and strengthen weak muscles to improve your overall shape. They are by no means intended to replace your chosen exercise programme or to form a short-cut to exercise. There isn't one in any case. But they are useful as a stop-gap, for example when you can't get to the gym or your regular class, or you want to top up your existing routine.

All these exercises are designed to be of minimal impact, particularly to the back and joints. Performed correctly, they should not put any strain on the back, neck or other joints and are therefore excellent for those people who suffer from related problems and are unable to participate in a regular exercise programme.

The exercises target the muscles in both the upper and lower body. In most people, the often underused inner thigh muscles need work. The lower calf exercise will improve the function of the plantar return reflex, and the abdominal exercises will aid posture and improve the function of the all-important thoraco-abdominal pump.

You will notice that there is no specific toning exercise included for the front thighs. This is because these muscles are already used frequently in everyday activities such as climbing stairs and running for the bus as well as in aerobic and step classes. Excessive use of these muscles may lead to dysmorphism, especially in people of a muscular build. However, it's always a good idea to stretch out and relax these commonly used muscles and, for this reason, I have included an appropriate stretch in the cool-down section.

Light weights and resistance bands may be used where recommended on the arms and legs. Resistance bands are wide strips of rubber-like material that provide some resistance to your muscular work, thus improving muscle tone and helping you burn more calories. They are available in several strengths, from the easy-to-pull to the quite resistant. The stronger the band, the harder the work will be, which means you will tire more easily and you may also build muscle bulk. Weights and bands can be purchased quite cheaply in most sports shops and sports sections of department stores.

Make sure you master the basic version of any exercise before attempting to use a band or weights.

If possible, practise these exercises in front of a mirror so that you can check your technique—although make sure the mirror is positioned in a suitable place so that you do not have to crane your neck to see yourself! The floor exercises should be performed on a well-cushioned floor or an exercise mat.

Do warm up before you start to help mobilise your joints and prepare your muscles for the work they will be undertaking. It's equally important to do some cool-down stretches afterwards to help prevent any muscle soreness. All stretches should be gently eased into, so do not bounce or try to push the body beyond its natural limits.

With the toning exercises you should do sufficient repetitions to ensure that the muscle you are working feels slightly fatigued, but not strained, as it is important to challenge the muscle if you are to see any progress. However, as with any exercise, if you feel any sharp or sudden pain you should stop immediately.

Let's go.

WARM UP

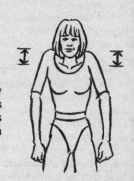

SHOULDER SHRUGS

Stand upright with feet comfortably apart, knees slightly bent and arms relaxed by your sides. Pull your shoulders up towards your ears, then relax them again. Repeat eight times.

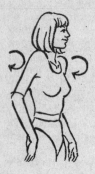

SHOULDER ROLLS

Roll both shoulders forwards eight times, then reverse the action and roll the shoulders backwards.

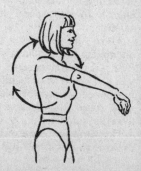

ARM CIRCLES

Now, exaggerate the movement and circle one elbow forwards eight times, then repeat with the other elbow. Repeat, circling the elbows backwards.

HIP CIRCLES

Keeping your knees slightly bent, place your hands on your hips and rotate the hips in a full circle. Do eight, then repeat in the opposite direction.

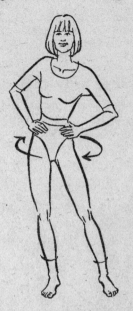

MARCHING

March on the spot, swinging your arms. Do sixteen.

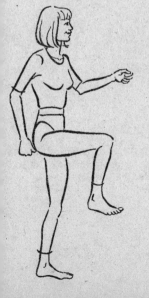

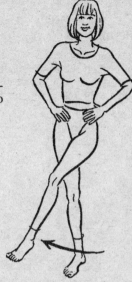

STEP AND KICK

Now step to the side and kick the opposite leg in front. Repeat sixteen times to alternate sides.

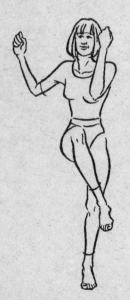

ELBOW TO KNEE

Lift each knee in turn and aim to touch the opposite elbow. Do sixteen with alternate knees.

MARCH

March on the spot again for sixteen counts.

WARM-UP STRETCHES

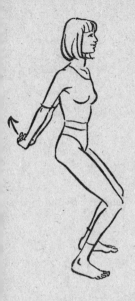

CHEST STRETCH

With feet hip-width apart and knees slightly bent, clasp your hands behind your back. Keep the elbows slightly bent. Slowly raise the arms as high as you can, and hold for a count of eight, then release

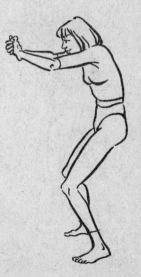

UPPER BACK STRETCH

Extend your arms in front at shoulder height and clasp the hands with palms facing outwards. Round your back and push forwards with the hands. Hold for a count of eight, then release.

SHOULDER STRETCH

Cross your right arm in front of your
chest and bring your left arm up, bent,
to hold your right arm against your
chest. Pull your left arm towards you,
pressing gently on the right elbow
while pushing away from the body with
the right arm. Hold for a count of eight,
then release.

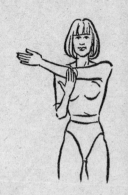

Change arms and repeat.

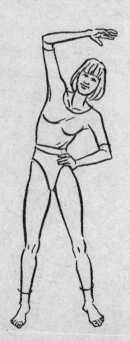

SIDE STRETCH

Stand with feet a comfortable dis-
tance apart and knees slightly
bent. Place your left hand on your
thigh for support and reach up and
over with your right arm, making
sure you lean directly to the side.
Hold for a count of eight, then
release.

Repeat to the other side.

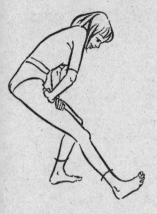

BACK THIGH (HAMSTRING) STRETCH

Bend your left knee and take your right foot out in front of you, resting your hands on your right thigh for balance. Keeping your neck and back straight, lean forwards and raise the toes off the floor. Feel the stretch in the back thigh of the extended leg. Hold for a count of eight, then release.

Repeat with the other leg in front.

CALF STRETCH

Stand with your left leg in front of your right leg. Keep both feet flat on the floor and slowly bend the front knee, making sure the knee bends over the ankle. Hold for a count of eight, then release.

Change legs and repeat.

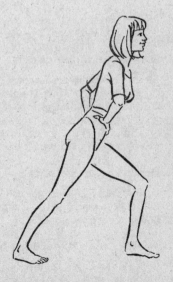

EXERCISES FOR THE BOTTOM, THIGHS AND CALVES

OUTER THIGHS

1 Basic

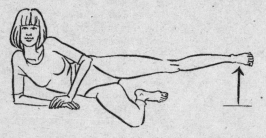

Lie on your side on the floor, keeping your hips square. Pull your tummy in. Place your other arm on the floor and bend your right leg to stabilise your torso.

Keeping your left leg straight, slowly lift it up to the count of eight, then slowly bring it down again. Repeat eight times.

Roll over and repeat on the other side.

2 Basic plus leg circles

Start in the same position as above.

Gently lift the right leg about 20 inches (50cm) off the floor. Keeping the ankle and foot relaxed, make small circles with the leg, first forwards then backwards.

Aim to do eight circles clockwise and eight anticlockwise, then roll over and repeat with the other leg.

3 Basic plus weights

Perform the basic exercises with light weights strapped to the ankles. Remember to make sure you have mastered the basic move before adding weights.

4 Basic plus resistance band

Perform the basic exercises with a band tied around your thighs. The lower down your legs you tie the band, the harder the thighs will have to work.

INNER THIGHS

1 Basic

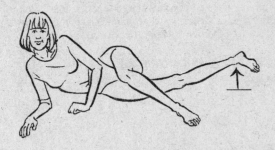

Lie on your right side, keeping your hips square. Bend your left leg and rest the foot on the floor in front so that your knee is off the floor.

Slowly lift your right leg about 12 inches (30cm) off the floor to a count of five. Hold in the air for five counts, then lower to a count of five. Repeat eight times. To ensure that you use only the inner thigh muscles, do not stretch or point the toes, but let the foot hang from the ankle.

Roll over and repeat on the other side.

2 Basic plus leg circles

Start in the same position as above and lift the leg about 12 inches (30cm) off the floor. Make small circles with the leg, keeping the movement slow and controlled. Remember to use only the inner thigh muscles. Repeat eight times.

Roll over and repeat on the other side.

3 Basic plus weights

Perform the basic exercises with light weights strapped to the ankles. Remember to make sure you have mastered the basic move before adding weights.

4 Basic plus resistance band

Perform the basic exercise with a band tied around your ankles.

Bottom

Lie face down on the floor and rest your head on your hands.
Clench the cheeks of your bottom together to a count of five, then
release. Imagine there is a dot on each cheek, and aim to pull these
as close together as possible. Repeat eight times.

Back thighs (hamstrings)
1 Basic

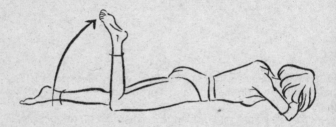

Lie face down on the floor and rest your head on your hands.
Clench your buttocks to tighten the muscles in your bottom.
Keeping the movement slow and controlled, bend your right knee
and lift the right foot off the floor until the calf is at right angles to
the thigh and the sole of the foot points towards the ceiling. You
should feel the hamstring muscle working. Slowly return the foot
to the floor. Repeat eight times.
    Repeat with the other leg.

2 Basic plus weights

Perform the basic exercise with light weights strapped to the
ankles.

3 Basic plus resistance band

Perform the basic exercise with a band tied around the ankle of the
stationary leg and the instep of the working foot.

CALF MUSCLES

Stand upright in a good posture with feet slightly apart and turned outwards slightly. Hold onto the back of a chair if necessary and slowly rise onto the balls of the feet to a count of three. Hold for a mount of three, then slowly lower your heels to the floor to a count of three. Repeat eight times.

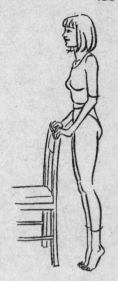

COOL-DOWN STRETCHES FOR THE LEGS

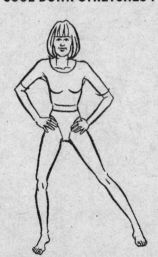

Inner thigh and calf stretch

Stand with feet wide apart and parallel so that the toes point forwards, and place your hands on your hips. Keeping your body upright, bend your right knee and keep the left leg straight. Feel the stretch in the left inner thigh. Hold for a count of sixteen, then release and return to the upright position.

Turn your body to the right and slide your feet as you turn so that you are now facing the right and your feet are still parallel. Bend the front (right) leg, ensuring the knee bends over

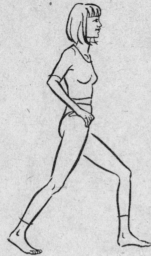

the ankle, and feel the stretch in the left calf. Make sure both heels remain on the floor. Hold for a count of sixteen, then release.

Return to the central position with legs apart and feet facing forwards, hands on hips. You are now ready to stretch on the other side.

Keeping the right leg straight, bend the left knee over the ankle and feel the stretch in the right inner thigh. Hold for a count of sixteen, then release.

Turn to the left, feet parallel and in line with your body. Bend the front (left) leg and feel the stretch in your right calf. Hold for a count of sixteen, then release and return to the central position.

FRONT THIGH (QUADRICEPS) STRETCH

Stand with feet together and hold onto the back of a chair with one hand. Bend one leg behind you and take hold of the foot (or heel) with your hand and gently pull the heel towards your bottom. Feel the stretch in the front of your thigh. Hold for a count of sixteen, then release.

Repeat with the other leg.

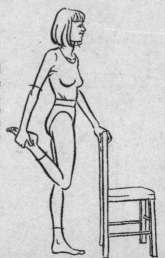

BACK THIGH (HAMSTRING) STRETCH

Standing upright, turn your left foot out slightly for balance. Take your right foot out in front of you, placing the foot flat on the floor and bend the left knee. Resting your hands on your right thigh for balance and keeping your neck and back straight, lean forwards and feel the stretch in the back thigh of the right leg. Hold for a count of eight, then release.

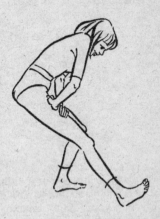

Repeat with the other leg in front.

EXERCISES FOR THE TUMMY AND BACK

TUMMY CURL

Lie on your back on the floor with knees bent and feet flat on the floor and place your hands on the front of your thighs. Pull your tummy muscles in—imagine your tummy button is trying to touch the small of your back. Now slowly raise your head, shoulders and ribcage off the floor, sliding your hands up your thighs as you lift. Take five counts to lift up, making sure your chin does not sink into your chest. Slowly return to the starting position on a count of five.

Repeat eight times, breathing out as you rise and breathing in as you lower.

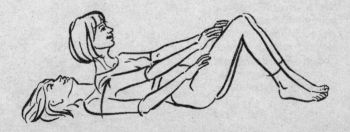

OBLIQUE CURL

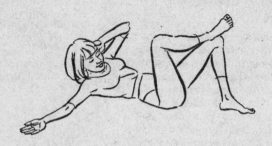

Lie on your back with knees bent, then place your left foot on your right knee. Place your right hand behind your head to support your neck and place your left arm out to the side on the floor.

Pull your tummy in and slowly raise your head, shoulder and ribcage off the floor, aiming your right shoulder towards your left knee. Count to three as you lift, then slowly return to the starting position on a count of three. Repeat eight times, breathing out as you lift and breathing in as you lower.

Change over arms and legs and repeat, aiming the left shoulder towards the right knee.

REVERSE CURL

Lie on your back with your arms by your sides, palms facing up. Bend your knees into your chest and cross your ankles. Breathe out and pull your tummy muscles in so that your hips move towards your ribcage. The knees will automatically come further towards your chest, but do not swing them in to assist. Repeat eight times.

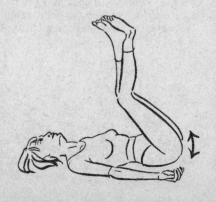

BACK STRENGTHENER

After working your tummy muscles it's important to do some back strengthening work.

Lie face down with hands loosely clasped and resting on your bottom. Slowly raise your upper body off the floor, then gently lower to the floor again. Repeat six times, breathing out as you lift and in as you lower.

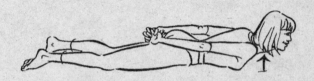

COOL-DOWN STRETCHES FOR THE TUMMY AND BACK

TUMMY STRETCH

Lie on your front with head and shoulders off the floor and support yourself on your forearms. Your elbows should be directly beneath your shoulders. Hold for a count of sixteen, then release.

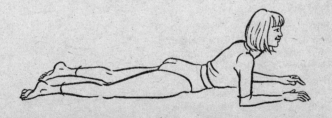

WAIST STRETCH

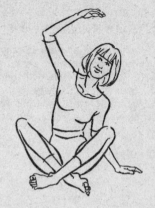

Sit cross-legged on the floor. Place one hand on the floor beside you and reach the other arm up and over your head. Keep both hips on the floor and feel the stretch in your waist. Hold for a count of sixteen, then release.

Repeat to the other side.

BACK STRETCH

Come up onto your knees, then lower your bottom onto your heels and lower your chest to the floor. Extend your arms in front on the floor as far as possible. Hold for a count of sixteen, feeling the stretch down your back.

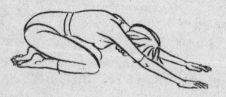

EXERCISES FOR THE ARMS, SHOULDERS AND CHEST

UPPER ARMS (BICEPS)

1 Basic

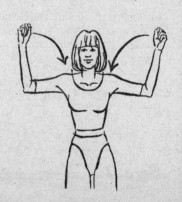

Stand upright with tummy in and legs slightly bent. Hold your arms out to the sides at shoulder height. Make loose fists with the hands.

Bend the arms at the elbows to bring the fists towards the

shoulders, then straighten the arms again. Perform each movement in a slow and controlled fashion. Repeat eight times.

2 Basic plus weights

Use light hand weights to increase the resistance of the exercises.

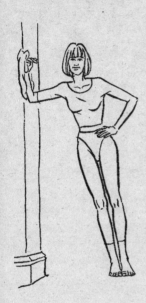

BACKS OF THE ARMS (TRICEPS)

This muscle easily becomes floppy, so here is a simple exercise that will help.

Find a soft cushion to protect your hands, or put socks over your hands. Stand sideways on to a wall and place your feet about 24 inches (60cm) away from the wall. Place the back of the hand and wrist against the wall, using the cushion for comfort, so that the elbow is bent and about 3 inches (7.5cm) away from the wall and your weight is supported on the back of the arm.

Gently move your upper body towards the wall, then push yourself back to the starting position. Repeat eight times, using slow and controlled movements, and feel the triceps muscle working.

Turn round and repeat with the other arm.

CHEST (PECTORALS)

1 Basic

Stand upright with tummy pulled in and place your arms out to the sides at shoulder height. Bend the arms and make loose fists with the hands.

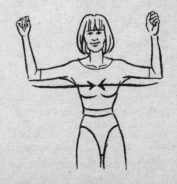

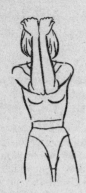

Keeping your elbows at shoulder height, bring the arms together to meet in front. Once the arms touch each other, take them out to the sides again. Repeat eight times.

2 Basic plus weights

Hold light weights in your hands to increase the resistance.

3 Basic plus resistance band

Place the band around your upper back and under the armpits and hold the ends with each hand.

SHOULDERS (DELTOIDS)

1 Basic

Stand upright with tummy pulled in and take your arms out to the sides at shoulder height, palms facing down.

Keeping the arms straight, raise them about 6 inches (15cm) and then bring them back down to shoulder height. Keep the movement slow and controlled. Repeat eight times.

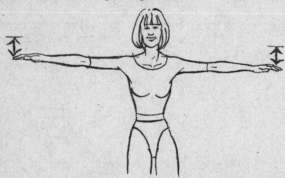

2 Basic plus arm circles

Keeping the arms outstretched, circle them forwards eight times, then backwards eight times. Keep the circles small (about 6 inches/15cm) in diameter.

3 Basic plus weights

You can hold light weights in your hands for either of the above shoulder exercises.

4 Basic plus resistance band

Place the band across your upper back and hold the ends with each hand.

SHOULDERS (RHOMBOIDS)

1 Basic

Stand with elbows pressed tight into your waist and your forearms in front with palms up. Keeping your elbows tight into your waist, take your forearms out to the sides. Now imagine there is a pencil between your shoulder blades. Pull your shoulders back as if you are trying to grasp the pencil between your shoulder blades. Relax and then bring the arms to the front again. Repeat eight times.

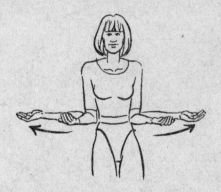

2 Basic plus weights

Hold light weights in each hand to increase the resistance.

3 Basic plus resistance band

Perform the first stage of the basic exercise with a band across your upper back and under your armpits, and hold onto the ends.

COOL-DOWN STRETCHES FOR THE ARMS, BACK, SHOULDERS AND CHEST

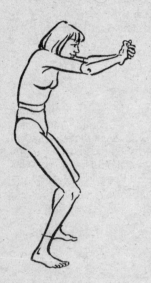

UPPER BACK STRETCH

Stand upright and extend your arms in front at shoulder height. Clasp the hands with palms facing outwards. Slowly round your back and push forwards with the hands as if trying to pull your shoulder blades apart. Hold for a count of sixteen, then release.

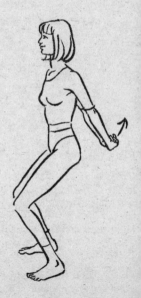

CHEST STRETCH

With feet hip-width apart and knees slightly bent, clasp your hands behind your back. Keep the elbows slightly bent. Slowly raise the arms as high as you can, pulling the shoulders back. Hold for a count of sixteen, then release.

SHOULDER STRETCH

Cross your right arm in front of your chest and bring your left arm up, bent, to hold your right arm against your chest. Pull your left arm towards you, pressing gently on the right elbow while pushing away from the body with the right arm. Hold for a count of sixteen, then release.
Change arms and repeat.

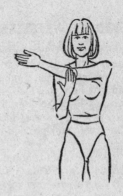

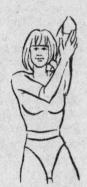

TRICEPS STRETCH

Bend your right arm and, with elbow pointing upwards, place the palm of the hand flat between your shoulder blades. Bring your left arm in front to press gently on the right elbow. Hold for six to ten seconds, then release.
Change arms and repeat.

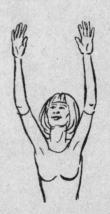

FULL BODY STRETCH

Extend both arms above your head as high as possible. Really feel as if you are reaching for the ceiling and feel the stretch down the whole of your body. Hold for a count of sixteen, then relax.

EVERYDAY EXERCISES TO TONE THE LEGS

An excellent way to improve the shape of the legs without acquiring muscle bulk is to perform weight-bearing exercises that stretch the muscles at the same time. Such exercises can easily be incorporated into your daily routine, whether you're at home, in the office, taking the dog for a walk or walking to the shops. You can also practise some of these exercises in the local swimming pool. The water will provide resistance and help you develop shapely legs.

1 Use the stairs at home or the office and go up them two or three steps at a time. This will both stretch and tone the muscles in front and back thighs and calves.

2 To work the outer and inner thighs, go up the stairs one at a time, but take wide steps so that you tread to either side of each step instead of in the middle.

3 Now on the flat, imagine you are jumping sideways over a puddle. Jump one foot to the side and follow with the other foot, pointing the feet as you jump. This works all the leg muscles and the plantar return reflex in the sole of the foot.

4 More on the puddle technique. Leap forwards and upwards with alternate legs as if jumping over a puddle, and feel the stretch and pull in the whole of your legs.

10

AROMATHERAPY, CREAMS, SUPPLEMENTS AND DRY SKIN BRUSHING

Aromatherapy, creams and other products and techniques can help treat cellulite if used in conjunction with other measures

AROMATHERAPY

- Aromatherapy is a powerful form of treatment for cellulite, providing the mixture is chosen correctly.
- Treatment must be applied locally (direct to the skin).
- It is recommended for all types of cellulite, in conjunction with other measures.

The use of plant extracts in healing is not new. Forty thousand years ago, the aborigine people used plants for their anti-infective, immune-boosting, stimulative and strengthening properties. Nowadays, there are advanced techniques which can determine the exact nature of chemical compounds found in plant tissue. Just about every part of the plant can be used – the roots, the leaves, the fruits and the buds – and many of these are effective in the treatment of cellulite and associated problems if used in conjunction with other methods. Different molecules can be extracted by different processes to obtain the desired effect: drying in air, freeze drying (leaves), extraction in alcohol, infusing in water or glycerine (buds) or distilling (essential oils).

Oils distilled from plants are known as essential oils and these are the ones used in aromatherapy. They are applied directly to the skin and are rapidly absorbed to reach first the underlying dermis and then the blood. Once absorbed, they affect many organs and are just as potent as conventional medicines; in fact, in high concentrations, they can be toxic. Pregnant women, in particular, need to take extra care as some oils can affect the foetus. Other oils are photosensitising; in other words they can cause a rash if the treated area is exposed to the sun. In many cases their use should be prescribed or at least supervised by a qualified practitioner. This is certainly the case on the Continent where the study and practice of aromatherapy extends far beyond the beauty therapy practice in the UK.

It is therefore advisable to consult a trained aromatherapist before attempting to treat yourself. However, aromatherapy kits specially designed for home use are now available to aid relaxation, wellbeing and so on, and these contain oils whose properties are known to be safe and reliable in the quantities given in the mixtures.

All oils should be diluted in a base oil, and the properties of the base oil often enhance the benefits of the aromatherapy mixture. Almond oil is commonly used as a base oil for massage purposes, but any mixtures that are directly applied to cellulite tissue should always contain hazelnut oil as the base oil as this has decongesting activities in its own right, unlike sweet almond oil.

Preferably after a bath or shower, apply the oil mixture. Drip a few drops onto the skin and then using gentle fan-like movements, rub into the skin, starting at the lowermost parts of the legs to be treated, moving upwards towards the heart. Only cover the areas that are troubled with cellulite. Rub gently and smoothly, always moving upwards with your movements. Remember that oils can stain your clothes, so it's always best to do this at night.

ESSENTIAL OILS IN THE TREATMENT OF CELLULITE

To be effective in the treatment of cellulite, essential oils need to have specific actions on the blood vessels, the fat cells and the lymphatic system.

Below is a list of essential oils that directly affect the veins, the lymph system, the microcirculation and the fat-releasing process itself. Some have been marked with an asterisk, and these are extremely potent oils whose effects extend far beyond the treatment of cellulite itself. Such oils, which interestingly enough are all lipolytic (fat-releasing), can be toxic to the foetus and must only be used if you are absolutely certain you are not pregnant. So do ask for professional advice before embarking on any home cure. If there is the slightest possibility that you are pregnant, it is essential that you avoid the use of these oils in your aromatherapy mixtures.

If you are planning to make up your own mixture, choose up to five constituent oils and measure them out exactly. It is best to use a small syringe to measure tiny quantities, and most hardware stores sell small plastic syringes. Throw away the syringe after use, as the plastic will absorb the oil that remains in the syringe and there is no reliable way of cleaning the syringe. Make sure you store the oils in a cool, dry place, otherwise they may become rancid.

Since essential oils are very potent you must take extreme caution during the mixing process. It's not like cooking, where if you add too much or too little of one ingredient it doesn't really matter. If you add too much or too little of any of the components in an aromatherapy mixture, then you may end up with a weak mixture or, worse still, a mixture that is too strong and irritating to the skin and body tissues. Again, if in doubt, consult a trained aromatherapist.

CHOOSING OILS

Remember to treat all underlying problems, including stress

When deciding which oils to include in your aromatherapy mixture, try to balance your selection so that it contains an oil suitable for improving venous function, one for improving lymphatic drainage, one for removing existing fluid retention and fibre formation and, if necessary, one for releasing fat. I would also recommend that you always include an oil that addresses the effects of stress on the body. "Beauty by Post" provides ready made oils and can make up clients' requirements as well as providing the base oils (see page 199 for address).

Choose up to five oils and then mix them in a sterilised dark glass jar or bottle. Use a maximum of 2ml of each oil, no more, then make up the mixture to 100ml by adding hazelnut oil (*Corylus avellana*) and shake well. To calculate how much hazelnut oil you need to add, use the following guide.

Number of oils in mixture	Amount of essential oil in mixture	Amount of hazelnut oil to add	Total
one	2ml	98ml	100ml
two	4ml	96ml	100ml
three	6ml	94ml	100ml
four	8ml	92ml	100ml
five	10ml	90ml	100ml

Essential oils of value in the treatment of cellulite

Essential oil	Common name	*Exclusions
Improving venous function		
*Cupressus sempervirens	evergreen cypress	breast disease
Juniperus mexicana	rock cedar	
Juniperus virginiana	red cedar	
Melaleuca alternifolia		
Valeriana wallichi	Cretan spikenard	
Cusparia trifoliata		

Decongesting (removing existing fluid and fibre formation)

Helichrysum italicum		
Juniperus mexicana	rock cedar	
Melaleuca cajeputii	cajeput	
Melaleuca quinquenervia	niaouli	

Improving lymph drainage		
Santalus album	sandalwood	
Cusparia trifoliata		
*Cedrus atlantica	Atlantic cedar	pregnancy
*Cedrus deodara	Indian cedar	pregnancy

Lipolytic (fat releasing)		
*Geranium macrorrhizum	geranium	pregnancy
*Cupressus arizonica	Arizonian cypress	pregnancy
*Salvia officinalis	sage	pregnancy
*Cedrus atlantica	Atlantic cedar	pregnancy
*Cedrus deodara	Indian cedar	
*Citrus limon	lemon	pregnancy

Regulator of the pituitary-ovarian axis
Very useful to include in an aromatherapy mixture if hormonal influences and gynaecological problems are a feature of the cellulite.

*Rosmarinus officinalis	rosemary	pregnancy

AROMATHERAPY MIXTURE FOR CELLULITE

This is my favourite, well-tested and reliable mixture for treating cellulite. Here, I am using six oils. Use two or three applications per day to the cellulite area. Rub gently into the skin, using your fingers and stroking upwards towards the heart. This mixture is not suitable for women who are pregnant or who suffer from breast disease.

Essential oil of Cupressus sempevirens (evergreen cypress)	2ml
Essential oil of Citrus limon	2ml
Essential oil of Cedrus atlantica (Atlantic cedar)	2ml
Essential oil of Salvia officinalis (sage)	2ml
Essential oil of Eucalyptus citriodora (eucalyptus)	2ml
Oil of Corylus avellana (hazelnut oil)	90ml

USING OILS TO TREAT ASSOCIATED PROBLEMS

Stress

Stress should never be overlooked as a potential cause and certainly as a promoter of cellulite. If you don't treat stress, then the cellulite may not shift as quickly as it ought to. Aromatherapy is an effective and extremely pleasant form of treatment.

Essential oil	Common name	Exclusions
Citrus reticulata		
Lavandula angustifolia	lavender	
Lippia citriodora	verbena	
Melissa officinalis	lemon balm	
Ocimum basilicum	basil	
Chamaemelum nobile	camomile	
*Citrus aurantium bergamia	bergamot	photosensitising
Leptospermum citratum	myrtle	
Eucalyptus citriodora	eucalyptus	

When making up these oils, use sweet almond oil as a base. Use up to three different components, adding 2ml of each and using a clean syringe to measure, and make up to 100ml with the sweet almond oil (see below). Remember always to use a sterilised, dark glass jar or bottle and shake well.

Number of oils in mixture	Amount of essential oil in mixture	Amount of sweet almond oil to add	Total
one	2ml	98ml	100ml
two	4ml	96ml	100ml
three	6ml	94ml	100ml

Aromatherapy mixture for stress

Here is my favourite aromatherapy mixture for treating stress.

Essential oil of Lavandula angustifolia (lavender)	2ml
Essential oil of Lippia citriodora (verbena)	2ml
Essential oil of Melissa officinalis (lemon balm)	2ml
Sweet almond oil	94ml

Neck pain

Using aromatherapy to relieve muscle pain and spasm in the neck will help treat cellulite found on the nape of the neck. Back and neck pain which result in the so-called Dowager's hump is often associated with a tiny deposition of cellulite on the neck, just over the painful area. This type of cellulite cannot be removed by the usual anti-cellulite measures, and it is necessary to treat the underlying cause.

Aromatherapy mixture for neck pain and cellulite on the nape of the neck

This mixture forms an excellent anti-inflammatory and muscle-relaxing solution. Apply it two to four times a day over the nape of the neck and the affected shoulder and neck muscles. It can also help relieve back pain. In this instance I'm using 8ml of camomile to ensure the mixture is a good muscle relaxant.

Essential oil of Chamaemelum nobile (camomile)	8ml
Essential oil of Laurus nobilis (bay)	2ml
Essential oil of Betula alleghaniensis (birch)	2ml
Essential oil of Lavandula angustifolium (lavender)	2ml
or Essential oil of Lippia citriodora (verbena)	2ml
Oil of Corylus avellana (relaxant and hazelnut oil for its decongesting properties)	86ml

ANTI-CELLULITE CREAMS

- There are many effective anti-cellulite creams on the market but they can be expensive.
- All creams are based on pharmaceutical products rather than natural plant products.
- Creams are useful for all types of cellulite except the well-advanced stages (stages five and six).

There is now a vast array of creams and gels available, many of which are useful in an anti-cellulite regime, but they do have their limitations. Except in the very early stages of cellulite development, in order to be effective, creams need to be used in conjunction with diet and exercise or medical treatment. Large areas of cellulite, heavily infiltrated by thick fibres, with poor circulation and huge steatomes, will simply not respond to creams alone. As a complementary therapy, though, they can be extremely beneficial. They improve the quality of the skin and prevent the development of further cellulite. Some creams, for instance BODI, have been specifically developed for use as an adjunct to medical treatment and for healing after surgery such as liposuction. Such creams, however, are of less value on their own, except in the very early stages of cellulite development.

Unlike aromatherapy mixtures, which are solely oil-based, creams consist of an emulsion of oil and water in varying quantities. Creams may be oil in water, giving a runny cream, or water in oil, which gives a thicker cream. The exact quantities of oil and water depend on the specific function of the cream and which active ingredients will be absorbed in it.

Gels, on the other hand, are water-based, and alcohol is often added as a drying and preserving agent. The active ingredient, for instance caffeine, must be water-soluble and the rate of absorption of the gel depends on its particular characteristics. The advantage of a cream over a gel is that both oil-soluble and water-soluble ingredients can be mixed together. Creams are also preferable for dry skins, but if you have a greasy skin you would be better off with a gel.

There are several substances used in cellulite creams and gels and the most effective ingredients are listed below. Many of these mixtures have been available on the Continent and some are now available in the UK. Any cream or gel will have to meet certain conditions before it can be considered useful in the treatment of cellulite. The active component must be stable in the mixture and survive storage at room temperature. It must also be able to pass through the thick outer layer of the skin, without being altered, to reach the affected tissues. Once in the tissues, it should remain there as long as possible. The active ingredients must not be toxic either to the skin or the general circulation and the mixture must not irritate the skin.

Creams that are lipolytic form a good adjunct to a weight-reducing diet or exercise regime, since they encourage the loss of fat from the areas to which they are applied and therefore can help counteract the action of the fat-storing receptors on the lower body. Such creams will contain one or more of the following ingredients: caffeine, aminophylline and silicium.

Decongestant creams are useful for treating heavy and water-logged legs with large areas of orange-peel skin, and anti-inflammatory creams will help treat heavy legs, broken veins, swollen ankles and improve the venous return.

Like most creams, all cellulite creams should be stored in a cool place and used up quickly to ensure that all the ingredients remain active. So, once you've bought a cream, don't store it away for months on end before using.

CHIEF COMPONENTS OF ANTI-CELLULITE CREAMS AND GELS

Choose creams wisely and beware of those that are marketed as "miracle" cures for cellulite. To make certain that the creams you choose will be effective, look for ones that contain the highest proportion of the following ingredients on the packaging.

Hedera helix·

An oil-based extract of ivy, Hedera helix has a decongesting effect on the tissues.

Centella asiatica

The extract of this wild chestnut plant is very useful in the treatment of cellulite. Once extracted, Centella asiatica can be used in both creams and tablets. It is also used in an injectable form by doctors for the treatment of cellulite by mesotherapy.

Centella asiatica has two important properties. First, it strengthens the walls of the veins, thus preventing them from damage or protecting against further damage in the case of veins that are already weakened. It also ensures that no further fluid leaks out uncontrollably into the tissues.

Centella asiatica also has a stimulating effect on the fibroblasts – the cells that create and repair tissue. One of the prime functions of these cells is to produce fine supporting fibres in between the fat cells whenever they are needed, for instance to repair damaged tissue after a cut or burn. Fibroblasts are sensitive cells, and lack of nutrients, in particular oxygen, makes them function abnormally and create thick, inelastic fibres that surround the fat cells and lead to the development of cellulite. Centella asiatica resolves this situation by making the fibroblasts more resistant to conditions of poor oxygenation and nutrient supply, and enabling them to function normally. Not only will they stop making thick, cellulitic fibres, but they will also start to reabsorb the abnormal fibres, ultimately replacing them with normal, finer, elastic, supportive ones.

Centella asiatica forms the basis of many creams both for cellulite and also for healing wounds. It is included in the cellulite creams BODI and Ecladerm. In its pure form it is sold as Madecassol.

Caffeine

Taken orally in moderate doses, caffeine increases the basal metabolic rate, but in higher doses it causes the small blood vessels to constrict, thus damaging the microcirculation and encouraging the development of cellulite. If it is applied directly to the skin, for instance in gel or cream form, it is rapidly absorbed to reach the subcutaneous tissue. This has the effect of stimulating the beta receptors on the surface of the fat cells and encouraging them to release fat into the bloodstream.

Aminophylline

This drug is normally used in the treatment of asthma and falls into the same category of chemicals as caffeine. Again, it stimulates the release of fatty acids into the bloodstream. Since aminophylline is less stable than caffeine and breaks down in the presence of heat, it must be stored in a cool place and used quickly.

Silicium

Silicium is an organic form of silica, a non-metallic element in the same chemical group as carbon. Silica, the inorganic form, is found in sand, glass and stone and does not have the same action as silicium.

Silicium has several different but complementary properties. It protects the small blood vessels, the microcirculation and ensures a good blood supply to the tissues, even when the tissues have developed cellulite. A good supply of blood through cellulite tissue will encourage the removal of cellulite. Like vitamins C and E, silicium protects the tissues and the microcirculation against the effects of free radicals. It also stimulates the beta receptors on the surface of the fat cells to aid the removal of fat.

Hazelnut oil (Corylus avellana)

Hazelnut oil has decongestive properties similar to Hedera helix. It also contains vitamin E which protects the body against the effects of free radicals.

Thiomucase

Thiomucase is an enzyme obtained from bulls' testicles (yes!) that acts on the thick fibres of mucopolysaccharides in cellulite tissue. As it passes through the tissue it breaks up the fibres and aids the penetration of other active substances. It is of particular value in congested tissue with large areas of orange-peel skin. Although it has a much stronger decongesting action than Hedera helix and hazelnut oil, it does not penetrate the skin as easily. In some cases thiomucase can cause an allergic rash, so it won't suit everyone.

L-carnitine

L-carnitine is an amino acid that transports free fatty acids into the mitochondria – the parts of the cells that are responsible for the burning of fat and sugar to provide energy – in other words the cell batteries. As for all other components of creams, providing it can cross the skin barrier, it will aid the fat-burning process in the areas to which the cream is applied.

TAGO-1

TAGO-1 is a mixture of super-oxygenated free fatty acids which block the toxic effects of arachidonic acid. Arachidonic acid is one of a number of toxic, destructive compounds formed in the veins as a result of local inflammation. Blocking the effects of arachidonic acid helps protect against further destruction by preventing fluid release and a build-up of toxic metabolites in the tissues.

TAGO–1 is a patented compound and is contained in the cellulite cream Cellulene, and is also in higher concentrations in Venoxyl, which is used to treat broken veins, heavy legs, swollen legs and leg ulcers.

PLANT PRODUCTS AVAILABLE IN SUPPLEMENT FORM FOR USE IN THE TREATMENT OF CELLULITE

- Supplements based on plant products are useful for advanced or stubborn cases of cellulite or when cellulite is widespread on the body.

CENTELLA ASIATICA

Recommended for:

- Advanced, tethered cellulite
- Widespread cellulite
- Cellulite on the upper arms
- Venous problems; fluid retention, congestion, broken veins

An extract of wild chestnut, Centella asiatica acts on the fibroblasts by stimulating the formation of normal collagen (fibrous tissue) and reducing the formation of abnormal collagen such as is found in cellulite tissue, cheloids (scar tissue) and scleroderma (collagen disease). It also strengthens the small veins. Centella asiatica is available as cream or supplements and is commonly used in mesotherapy.

The recommended dosage for supplements is six tablets of 100mg every day. It is well tolerated by the body and there are virtually no side effects, which means it can be taken over a long period of time. It is particularly useful in advanced cases of cellulite where the legs have been heavily infiltrated with fibres, fat and fluid, and in cases where the cellulite is widespread over other parts of the body such as the arms, tummy and bottom.

SEAWEEDS (KELP AND FUCUS)

Recommended for:

- Congested tissues
- Weight problems
- Constipation

Seaweed contains iodine which, when taken orally, helps stimulate the thyroid gland. The thyroid gland is responsible for regulating the metabolic rate – the rate at which the body uses calories.

Kelp and fucus are brown seaweeds that contain mucilage, a gluey substance that acts as a decongestant when taken orally. The mucilage tends to remove excess body fluid, which is particularly helpful in cases of fluid-filled cellulite tissue. It also aids the passage of foods through the intestines, thus helping to treat constipation, abdominal bloating and digestive problems.

Kelp or fucus supplements must be taken with plenty of water. Iodine can be toxic in high doses, so never exceed the recommended dose.

GINKGO BILOBA

Recommended for:

- Poor veins; fluid retention; heavy legs
- Easy bruising

Ginkgo biloba is a tree indigenous to China, but it is now also found in many parks and large gardens in the UK. Ginkgo biloba contains the active components, Ginkgo heterosides, which strengthen the small veins and arteries. If you have poor circulation and weak veins – easy bruising, heavy legs and broken veins are probably the most obvious indications – Ginkgo biloba is a good supplement to take. In some ways, Ginkgo biloba is similar to Centella asiatica in that it strengthens the small veins but, unlike Centella asiatica, it has no beneficial effect on the fibroblasts.

There is no recommended daily dosage, so follow the instructions indicated on the packet.

VITIS VINIFERA (RED GRAPE, GRAPE VINE)

Recommended for:

- Poor veins; fluid retention; heavy legs
- Easy bruising
- Poor circulation

Extracts of the noble grape, the leaves, skins and bark give Vitis vinifera, commonly known as red grape or grapevine. Red grape contains flavonoids and tannins that strengthen the walls of the small veins and lymphatics, thus improving the return of blood from the legs. The reason why red wine in moderate doses is beneficial to the microcirculation is due to the tannin in the skins of the grapes rather than the alcohol itself. Red grape is available as a dried extract in supplement form and is useful for heavy legs, broken veins, discoloured skin resulting from broken veins and, of course, cellulite. Follow the recommended dosage on the packet.

ARTICHOKE (CYNARA SCOLYMUS)

Recommended for:

- Weight problems
- Constipation
- Fluid retention
- Fatty areas on the legs, hips and thighs

Artichoke, or Cynara scolymus, is a wonderful plant to use in the treatment of cellulite as it has many beneficial effects, so aim to include it regularly in your diet. Its stimulative effect on the intestines makes it a useful aid for treating constipation by helping the removal of toxins. It stimulates the liver, thus helping to release waste products held within the liver tissue, and it acts as a diuretic by removing excess fluid from the tissues. Artichoke also promotes the removal of fat from the fat cells and should therefore form an essential component of any weight-reducing regime.

Artichoke is available as Cynara scolymus in supplement form from health food stores and from pharmacies. Too much artichoke, however, particularly in tablet form (it's not easy to eat too many whole artichokes!), can cause diarrhoea, so you'll soon know if you've taken too much.

When starting a course of Cynara supplements, the first thing that will happen is a huge release of waste products from the liver, and in some cases this may overload the small ducts that empty the liver. In some people, this could cause liver spasm and a feeling of discomfort in the abdomen. This should pass as the backlog of toxins is dealt with, but if you should suffer any prolonged abdominal pain as a result of taking Cynara, then you should reduce the dosage and, if necessary, consult your doctor. Once Cynara has started to work, however, the liver drains its toxins easily. If you suspect that your liver is a little bit lazy or you have a particular liver or gall bladder problem such as gallstones, then start on a very small dosage and work up.

Cynara scolymus can also be extracted and purified to give a solution that is used by doctors in injections. In its injected form it is used on the Continent for the treatment of liver problems. However, its detoxifying actions, its diuretic (fluid-removing) and lipolytic properties also make it a wonderful preparation for the treatment of cellulite if injected directly into the affected tissues as in mesotherapy.

HORSETAIL (EQUISETUM)

Recommended for:

- Poor circulation
- Weak veins
- Tethered tissues

Horsetails are green plants that grow in bogs and marshes and are closely related to ferns. Their stems are reinforced with silica, which helps them stand up firmly in a wet, semi-solid environment. Silica, in its inorganic form, is found in glass, sand, rock – and of course, computer chips – and is of no use to the human body. However, the silica found in plants, most commonly in the horsetail plant, is organic and known as silicium which is well absorbed by the body. Indeed, it is now recognised as an essential trace element.

Silicium strengthens the walls of the small arteries and veins and also helps repair the lining of arteries that have been damaged by free radicals and cholesterol.

Silica, in its inorganic form, is also diluted and used by homeopathic practitioners to treat disorders of the circulation, particularly chilblains and vasculitis (inflammation of the small vessel walls).

Silicium can therefore be extremely beneficial in the treatment of cellulite and heavy legs, and is available in supplement form as extract of horsetail (Equisetum). Extract of horsetail is remarkably non-toxic. Nevertheless, you should always follow the manufacturer's instructions for dosage. Silicium can also be injected directly into cellulite tissue, and is commonly used in mesotherapy techniques.

Interestingly, silicium has recently become available for use in the treatment of hair loss. It works on the same principle of improving blood supply to the scalp. We shall no doubt see more and more uses of silicium in the next few years.

DRY SKIN BRUSHING

- A useful home remedy best combined with the use of an anti-cellulite cream or aromatherapy.
- Useful for all types of cellulite.
- Improves the skin texture rather than decreasing the volume of cellulite.

The aim of dry skin brushing is to stimulate the lymphatic drainage and improve the circulation. It's a technique that is easily acquired and involves gently brushing the skin with a special brush, designed to be used dry so that it does not pull on the skin.

Dry skin brushing should be a pleasant experience and should take only five to ten minutes. Aim to do it every day. The best time to do it is after a bath when you are warm, relaxed and in no hurry. Start at the ankles, using gentle, fan-like movements, and work up to the thighs and beyond to the bottom if necessary. It is important to keep the movements gentle, even though the temptation is to pummel the cellulite with the intention of "breaking it up." Breaking it up, however, would damage the delicate lymph vessels and microcirculation and certainly would not help your cellulite.

Follow the brushing by gently applying an anti-cellulite cream or aromatherapy mixture. The improvement in lymphatic drainage and microcirculation will help the action of the oil.

Dry skin brushing will improve the texture and appearance of the skin and is thus recommended for all types of cellulite. However, used alone, it is unlikely to reduce the volume. Applying an anti-cellulite cream that stimulates the release of fat (for example, aminophylline or caffeine), or a lipolytic aromatherapy mixture, after your skin brushing session may well result in some reduction in the volume of your cellulite. Again, be realistic. Huge steatomes, or fluid-filled legs with large swollen veins will need a far more powerful method and you may need professional help.

GLOSSARY OF TERMS

abdomen
The area of the body that lies between the chest and pelvis and contains the abdominal organs.

acesulfame K
An artificial sweetener.

acupressure
Medical technique akin to acupuncture, using pressure instead of needles to stimulate the acupuncture points.

acupuncture
A medical technique originating from China that involves the application of needles to certain points of the body.

adhesions
Abnormal fibrous tissue that may develop within any body cavity, in particular the abdomen or pelvis, after surgery or inflammation.

adrenal glands
A pair of glands that lie in the body above each kidney and are responsible for the secretion of adrenaline.

adrenaline
Hormone made by the adrenal glands and released into the blood under conditions of stress, fright or threat to give the body an energy boost in order to run away or to fight back.

Alexander technique
A technique aimed at correcting postural problems.

Allergy
Abnormal overreaction by the body's immune system to a harmless substance, for example hay fever is the abnormal reaction of the body to pollen.

alpha linolenic acid
One of the essential fatty acids.

alpha-2 receptor
Area on the surface of the fat cell that allows fat storage.

aminophylline
Drug normally used for treating asthma that has fat-releasing properties when applied directly to fatty tissue.

ampoule
Small glass vial or container containing medicine.

anaphylactic shock
Life-threatening allergic reaction in the body.

anti-inflammatory
Any substance that can reduce inflammation in the body.

antioxidants
Substances that prevent harmful degradation of food (as in food additives) and of cell components in the body (as in vitamins).

arachidonic acid
Toxic substance released by the walls of the veins when damaged, for instance by back-pressure of venous blood.

arteriole
Medium sized blood vessel leading from an artery to a capillary, carrying oxygenated blood.

arteriosclerosis
Medical terminology for "hardening of the arteries," a condition that develops with advancing age and can lead to heart disease and poor circulation.

aspartame
An artificial sweetener.

artery
Large blood vessel that carries blood from the heart to the body.

basal metabolic rate
The rate at which the body uses up energy at rest.

beta-carotene
Antioxidant vitamin that is changed in the body to vitamin A. Found mostly in carrots, tomatoes and coloured vegetables.

beta-receptor
Area on the surface of the fat cell that allows the release of fat.

biceps
Muscle at the front of the upper arm that flexes the arm at the elbow.

bile duct
Tube leading from the gall bladder into the duodenum carrying bile.

body mass index
A measurement of body weight expressed as a relàtion to height.

bowel flora
Bacteria that inhabit, quite normally, the intestines.

calipers
Instrument for measuring the thickness of skin.

candidiasis
Condition that arises due to infection of the body with Candida albicans, a yeast that causes thrush.

capillary
Small blood vessel that flows from the arterioles and penetrates deep into the tissues.

carbohydrate
Foodstuff such as sugar and starch used by the body for energy production.

carbon dioxide
Waste gas formed in the body as a result of energy production and expelled in the breath.

cassava
Foodstuff commonly eaten by some ethnic communities, related to arrowroot. Also known as manioc or gari.

cell
The basic unit of tissue, surrounded by a membrane and containing components for metabolism.

cellulite
Medical condition that is due to development of abnormal fibres and water retention amongst fatty subcutaneous tissue.

cellulolipolysis
Medical technique for treating cellulite, involving the placing of long fine needles under the skin and passing a gentle electric current through them.

cellulose
Indigestible fibre found in vegetables and pulses.

Centella asiatica
Plant that gives rise to an extract of the same name used in the treatment of cellulite.

chelate
Chemical term meaning bind with and remove, normally unwanted and toxic substances.

cheloid
Abnormal overgrowth of scar tissue after injury or operation found in certain individuals.

chiropractic
Medical technique involving manipulation of the spine and joints to treat back and neck pain.

cholesterol
Fatty substance found in animal products that can build up and block the arteries causing the heart and blood-vessel disease known as arteriosclerosis.

chromium
Metallic element necessary in small quantities in the body used in the metabolism of sugar.

chronic
Continuing for a long time.

cobalt
Metallic element necessary in very small quantities used in the treatment of sugar craving, also used by the cells for the removal of fat.

colitis
Medical term to describe inflammation of the colon (part of the large intestine).

collagen
Fibrous, supportive substance found most commonly in body tissues. Used for support of organs, skin, etc.

colon
Another word for the first part of the large intestine.

colonic irrigation
Specialised treatment that involves the removal of bowel contents by a tube inserted via the anus, after which the colon is then washed clean with water. Performed in a clinic by specially trained therapist.

complex carbohydrate
Large, complex sugar or starch molecule that takes a long time to digest.

congested
Full (of fluid, blood).

cranial osteopathy
Osteopathic treatment specifically applied to the head.

degenerative disease
Progressive disease associated with the ageing of the body, for example osteoarthritis.

deltoid
Muscle that covers the shoulder joint and lifts the arm upwards and outwards.

deoxygenated
No longer containing oxygen.

diaphragm
The muscle that lies between chest and abdomen that assists in breathing.

diathermy
Application of an electric current to seal, burn or remove the desired tissues. Also technique used in sealing broken veins; diathermy current given via fine needle into the veins.

diuretic
Substance that promotes removal of fluid from the body by stimulating the kidneys. Mostly prescribed medicine but naturally occurring diuretics also available.

Doppler
A non-invasive medical investigation to show the rate of flow of fluids through the body.

Dowager's hump
Colloquial term for the lump on back of neck often found in women, associated with neck and shoulder pain.

duodenum
The beginning of the small intestine that leads from the stomach.

dysfunction
Abnormal function.

dysmorphism
Medical term that refers to the fluid and fat-filled tissue that lies over the front of the thighs, often associated with exercise, also found in men.

echography
Medical investigation to demonstrate structure of specific areas of the body, similar to X-ray.

eczema
Skin disease, often allergic in origin, with dry, itchy, sometimes weepy, irritated areas of skin.

eicosapentanoic acid (EPA)
Oil found naturally in oily fish that protects against heart disease and inflammation.

emulsifier
Substance that allows oils and water to mix and remain stable.

emulsion
A mixture of liquids not soluble in each other; one being finely dispersed in the other. For example, oil in a water-based cream.

endorphin
Substance released by the brain to reduce pain in the body and induce a feeling of wellbeing and relaxation.

enzyme
Naturally occurring protein that speeds up physiological processes in the body, for example digestion of foods, creation of new body tissues and removal of toxins.

essential fatty acids
Naturally occurring fats that are necessary for the function of the body but cannot be made by the body and therefore need to be obtained from dietary sources.

faeces
Waste products of digestion stored in the rectum.

fallopian tubes
The tubes leading from the ovaries to the uterus (womb) carrying the ovum (egg).

faradism
Muscle toning and strengthening technique whereby muscles of the body are stimulated by a gentle electrical current applied via pads attached to the skin, sometimes combined with ionothermie.

fatty acid
The form in which fat is carried in the blood.

femoral artery
Large artery carrying oxygenated blood from the pelvis to the legs.

femoral vein
Large vein carrying deoxygenated blood back from the legs to the pelvis.

fibroblast
Specialised cells in body that create, remove and regulate structural fibrous tissue in the body. Responsible for the structure-forming collagen and elastin found amongst all tissues, also for repair of tissue in the healing process.

fibrous tissue
Tough, inelastic tissue like gristle that is formed by fibroblasts.

flavonoids
Vitamin-like substances found in fruits and vegetables that protect the body against damage by free radicals.

foetus
Unborn baby developing in womb.

follicle stimulating hormone (FSH)
Hormone released by the pituitary gland in the brain that sends messages to the ovary.

free radical
Highly charged thus toxic oxygen molecule produced in the body as a result of the action of chemicals, smoking and sun which damage cell components.

fructose
Sugar found in fruit.

Fucus
Generic name for certain seaweeds.

Fungi
Botanical term for mushrooms.

Fybogel
Medical product containing non-wheat fibre for the treatment of constipation.

Galactozyme
Trade mark for product that aids bloating and wind by digesting cellulose in the diet.

gall bladder
Pear-shaped gland that lies just under the liver and stores bile.

gamma linolenic acid
One of the essential fatty acids.

gari
Another name for cassava or manioc.

Ginkgo biloba
Ancient Chinese plant whose extract is useful in the treatment of weak veins.

glandular fever
Infectious viral disease caused by the Epstein-Barr virus that produces fatigue, malaise, sore throat and swollen lymph glands.

glucose
Sugar molecule.

glucose tolerance factor
Chromium in an organic form available as nutritional supplements to aid insulin and its action on sugar control.

glycogen
Storage form of carbohydrates including sugar found in the liver and muscles.

gynaecological
Pertaining to the female reproductive system.

Hedera helix
Botanical name for Ivy. Extract of Hedera Helix has decongesting properties.

hives
Common name for urticaria.

homeopathy
Medical treatment that uses dilutions of active substances as remedies, the choice of treatment being related not only to the nature and symptoms of the disease but also the characteristics of the sufferer. The dilution chosen to treat the disease mirrors the effects of the undiluted substance on a healthy body.

homogenous
In medical terms, of the same texture.

hormone
Chemical substance made by glands in the body that travels in the blood to carry messages from one gland to one or more.

hormone replacement therapy (HRT)
Treatment of the menopause by small doses of female hormone.

Horsetail
Plant that contains a lot of silicium. Silicium protects tissues from free radical damage, stimulates fat-release from fat cells and stimulates the microcirculation.

hyperaemia
Medical term for excess blood supply to part of the body, for example, the skin.

hypoglycaemia
Medical term for low blood sugar.

immune system
Bodily system of white blood cells that protect against disease. White blood cells may directly destroy invading micro-organisms or indirectly by producing antibodies.

infiltration
Process of entering amongst the tissues.

inflammation
Swelling, pain, redness and heat caused by tissue reaction to bacteria, viruses or other noxious stimulus.

inguinal canal
Tight anatomical channel at top of thigh that houses blood and lymph vessels supplying and draining the legs.

inorganic
In chemical terms, not associated with the carbon atom. Simpler molecule but in general more difficult to be absorbed by the body.

inspiration
Biological term for breathing in.

insulin
Hormone released from the pancreas into the blood to regulate blood sugar.

intravenous
Given directly into the vein by injection.

iodine
Non-metallic element necessary for the functioning of the thyroid gland.

ion
Element with an electrical charge; element in a chemically reactive form.

ionothermie
Method of treating cellulite by the application of clay-based paste to the legs.

irritable bowel syndrome
Disorder of the intestines causing pain, bloating, constipation and/or diarrhoea.

Isogel
Preparation of non-wheat fibre for the relief of constipation.

kelp
Type of seaweed used as nutritional supplement, rich in iodine.

L-carnitine
Carnitine is a protein substance found in the body that facilitates the breakdown of fat. Available as synthetic L-carnitine, found in some anti-cellulite creams.

lactic acid
Waste product of anaerobic exercise produced by muscle tissue.

Lactobacillus
Specially cultured bacteria that aid the normal bowel flora.

large intestine
The large digestive organ that is tube shaped, lies in the pelvis and joins onto the rectum.

leg ulcer
Medical condition caused by lack of blood to the legs resulting in non-healing, often infected, open area.

ligament
Tough fibrous tissue that attaches bones to other bones.

linoleic acid
One of the essential fatty acids.

lipolysis
Removal of fat from fat cell.

lipolytic
Having the ability to remove fat from fat cells.

liposculpture
The removal of fat from fatty deposits under the skin by inserting a small tube and sucking out the excess fat. Performed under local anaesthetic.

liposuction
The removal of fat from fatty deposits under the skin by inserting a tube at operation and sucking out the excess fat. Performed under general anaesthetic.

lordosis
Medical term for excess curvature of the small of the back.

lumbar
Pertaining to the region of the lower part of the back.

leuteinising hormone (LH)
Hormone released by the pituitary gland in the brain that stimulates the ovary.

lymph
Protein-rich fluid that escapes from the blood to enter the tissues and bathe the cells of the body, supplying them with nutrients and oxygen.

lymph node
Nodule of tissue situated at various intervals along the lymph channels

that contains many white cells to clean the lymph fluid before its return to the blood.

lymph vessels
The fine tubes along which lymph fluid flows.

lymphangiogram
Medical investigation to demonstrate the structure and flow of lymph vessels on X-ray.

lymphatic
Referring to the lymph system.

lymphoedema
A medical condition involving abnormal swelling due to retention of lymph fluid, usually in the legs or arms.

magnesium
Metallic element used in the body for many processes.

manganese
Metallic element required by the body in small quantities. Has a role in releasing fat from fat cells.

manioc
Another word for Cassava or gari.

Manual Lymphatic Drainage
Massage technique devised for stimulating the return of lymph from the tissues to the general circulation.

mattress skin
Common term for the appearance of well established, puckered, tethered cellulite.

membrane
The outer covering layer of a cell.

mesotherapy
Medical technique of French origin that involves giving tiny amounts of medicine at the site of disease by injection just under the skin.

metabolism
The underlying energy-giving, growth and repair mechanism of the body.

metabolite
Unwanted, often toxic, product of cell metabolism.

microcirculation
The capillary system that supplies the tissues with oxygenated blood.

mitochondria
Energy-producing part of the cell.

monosodium glutamate
Flavour enhancer used in packaged and Chinese food.

morphine
Medical substance that removes pain and creates a feeling of wellbeing. Used in the treatment of severe pain. Can be addictive.

mucilage
Gluey, gelatinous substance found in some foods that aids the passage of faeces through the intestines.

mucopolysaccharide
Thick fibrous substance made from protein and starch in the body; precursor to fibrous tissue itself.

nickel
Metallic element needed by the body in small amounts for sugar metabolism.

nodular
Full of nodules; lumpy bumpy.

non-hormonal
Not based on hormones.

oestrogen
Female hormone secreted by the ovary that affects female sex organs, skin, bones, blood vessels and all parts of the female body.

oligoelement
Another word for mineral needed by the body in small quantities. Also known as trace element.

oligotherapy
French medical treatment that uses small amounts of trace minerals to treat various disorders.

orange peel
Term used to describe the appearance of skin that has been swollen by fluid trapped in the tissues.

organic
In chemical terms, based on or containing the carbon atom. Organic compounds of, for example, metals are easily absorbed and utilised by the body.

osteopath
Practitioner who is trained in the manipulation of bones, ligaments,

muscles and joints to relieve back and neck pain and other muscular and bony complaints.

ovarian-pituitary axis
The hormonal relationship between the ovaries in the pelvis and the pituitary gland in the brain.

ovary
Glands occurring in pairs in the female pelvis close to the uterus that secretes oestrogen and progesterone and makes an ovum (egg) every four weeks in preparation for pregnancy.

oxygenated
With oxygen, for example, blood.

pancreas
Single gland that lies against the back wall of the abdomen and secretes insulin to regulate sugar level. Also secretes many digestive juices into the duodenum.

pectoral muscles
Muscle across each side of the chest, under the breast.

pelvic inflammatory disease
Medical term for inflammation of the gynaecological organs.

pelvis
The bony basin-like structure that lies at the base of the spine and contains and protects the organs of the pelvis.

photosensitiser
Substance that if applied to the skin will provoke a rash when exposed to the sun or ultraviolet light.

physiological
Referring to the natural processes of the body.

Pilates
Exercise technique that improves posture and tones specific muscles.

pituitary gland
Gland situated in the brain that controls the functioning of all other glands in the body, for example the ovaries, thyroid.

plantar fascia
The thick band of fibrous tissue that lies across the base of the foot from the heel to the toes.

plantar return reflex
The reflex action that stimulates return of lymph from the legs that is

brought about by the stretching of the plantar fascia, as in for example, dancing.

plaque
Medical term for build-up of hard, unwanted substance inside the arteries that leads to arteriosclerosis.

plasma
The fluid within the blood in which is dissolved nutrients, glucose and hormones.

platelet
One of the blood cells that is involved in the clotting of blood.

polarity
The electrical charge or activity across a cell membrane.

polysaccharide
A carbohydrate made from many simple sugars joined together in a chain.

potassium
A metallic element necessary for the functioning of the body most commonly found in vegetables and fruits.

procaine
Medical substance originally used as local anaesthetic, now used in mesotherapy for its vasodilating effects.

progesterone
One of the female hormones secreted by the ovaries.

protein
Naturally occurring compound made up of carbon, hydrogen, oxygen and nitrogen that forms the basis of body tissue, muscle, skin, blood, etc.

quadriceps
Large muscle at the front of each thigh.

receptor
A microscopic area on the cell surface that allows the passage of substances in and out of the cell.

red blood cell
One of the blood cells. Carries oxygen around the body in the blood.

respiration
In common terms, the act of breathing. More correctly, the process that occurs in the cells in order to provide energy for the cell.

rhomboids
One of a group of muscles binding the shoulder blades to the spine.

rutin
Plant extract that strengthens veins.

saccharin
An artificial sweetener.

salpingitis
Medical term for infection or inflammation of the fallopian tubes of the uterus.

scleroderma
Disease of excess collagen production that affects mostly the skin and the blood vessels, making them hardened and thickened. Also known as systemic sclerosis.

sclerosing
Any substance that irritates or hardens certain tissues in particular veins and destroys them.

sclerotherapy
Medical removal of broken veins by the injection into the vein of sclerosing agent.

secrete
A scientific term meaning produce and then release.

silica
Non-metallic element necessary for the healthy functioning of the circulation, also involved with fat release from fat cells.

silicium
An organic form of silica that is well absorbed by the body and used to create healthy tissues.

small intestine
The first part of the intestine leading from the stomach. Fat absorption occurs here. The small intestine leads on to the large intestine.

sodium
A metallic element necessary for the normal water balance and functioning of the body. Found most commonly in salt (sodium chloride).

sorbitol
An artificial sweetener.

stasis
Medical term for standstill; not moving.

steatome
Word derived from the French, referring to the large fatty areas surrounded by fibres found in cellulite.

sterilisation
Operation that involves cutting or burning of the fallopian tubes to prevent pregnancy.

stimulant
Any substance that stimulates the body, stimulating thought, heart rate, activity or other processes.

subcutaneous
Lying beneath the skin.

sublingual
Beneath the tongue.

TAGO-1
Patented solution available in Cellulene cream for the treatment of heavy veins and cellulite. Acts to block the effect of arachidonic acid that is released by inflammation of the vein walls, the inflammation invariably caused by stasis of blood.

tannins
Naturally occurring substances that strengthen the veins, found in tea, grapes and red wine.

tissue
Collection of cells with the same shape and function: for example fatty tissue, liver tissue.

Therapeutic massage
Specific massage technique particularly for the relief of back and neck problems.

thermal imaging
Non-invasive medical technique that identifies difference in temperature across a skin surface.

thiomucase
Enzyme used in medicine for removal of excess tissue fluid and breakdown of abnormal fibres.

thoraco-abdominal pump
The pumping action that the diaphragm has on the venous blood and lymph as it ascends and descends in the thorax during the process of breathing.

thorax
The chest.

thrush
Common name for infection of the mouth, vagina, etc, with the yeast Candida albicans.

thyroid gland
Gland in the neck that secretes thyroxine and controls the rate at which body functions (metabolism).

thyroxine
Hormone release by the thyroid gland. Controls metabolism, heart rate and other body processes, stimulates fat release from fat cells.

toxin
Potentially harmful product or chemical.

trace element
Element necessary for the body in very small quantities. Also called oligoelement.

triceps
Muscle at the back of each upper arm that extends the arm at the elbow.

TVP
Textured vegetable protein, normally produced from soya.

ultrasound
Medical investigation whereby sound waves are bounced off parts of the body and are reflected back and shown on to a screen. Demonstrates the shape, size and nature of underlying tissues.

urticaria
Medical term for rash of the skin that is characterised by raised itchy blotches. Commonly known as hives. Usually caused by an allergy.

uterus
The womb. Organ in the pelvis that receives the egg and, if fertilised, allows the development of a foetus.

varicose eczema
Skin rash arising at the ankles associated with varicose veins.

varicose ulcer
Open, non-healing area of skin on the lower leg due to congested legs and poor venous function associated with varicose veins.

varicose vein
Abnormally swollen vein visible just under the skin on the legs.

vasculitis
Medical term for inflammation of the small blood vessels.

vasoconstrict
The constriction (getting narrower) of a blood vessel in the body.

vasoconstrictor
A substance that makes a blood vessel in the body constrict (get narrower).

vasodilate
The widening (dilation) of a blood vessel in the body.

vasodilator
Any substance that will widen (dilate) a blood vessel.

vein
A blood vessel that returns blood from the body to the heart. In the tissues, veins carry away waste products and carbon dioxide.

venous
Pertaining to the veins.

venule
A small vein.

vertebra
Any of the bones making up the back; the cervical, thoracic and lumbar. The sacrum is made up of five fused vertebrae.

vessel
In medical terms, a tube. For example, lymph vessel, blood vessel.

Vodder technique
The Manual Lymphatic Drainage technique described by Dr Emil Vodder and his wife in the 1930s.

white blood cell
One of the blood cells that is responsible for the protection of the body against infection.

yo-yo diet
Going on and off diets, following a diet, losing weight and then eating again only to regain the weight lost.

zinc
Metallic element necessary for tissue healing, growth and sugar metabolism in the body.

FURTHER READING

The Bottom Line, Karen Amen, Vermilion.

The Complete Guide to Food Allergy and Intolerance, Dr. Jonathan Brostoff and Linda Gamlin, Bloomsbury.

The Crunch, Karen Amen with Tee Dobinson, Vermilion.

Food Combining for Health: a New Look at the Hay System, Doris Grant and Jean Joice, Thorsons.

McCance and Widdowson's The Composition of Foods, A.A. Paul and D.A.T. Southgate, HMSO Publications.

Nutritional Medicine, Dr. Stephen Davies and Dr. Alan Stewart, Pan Books.

Pottenger's Cats: A Study in Nutrition, Francis M. Pottenger, Jr., MD, Price-Pottenger Nutrition Foundation, Inc.

Raw Energy, Leslie and Susannah Kenton, Vermilion.

The Reebok Ultimate Guide to Fitness, Chantal Gosselin, Vermilion.

The Vital Vitamin Fact File, Dr. H. Winter Griffith, Thorsons.

Useful Addresses

Anti-cellulite creams and ready-made aromatherapy mixtures

Beauty by Post
50A High Street
Poole
Dorset
BH15 1BT
Tel: 01249 819160

Information and products; food and environmental allergies

The Allergy Shop Ltd
PO Box 196
Haywards Heath
West Sussex
RH16 3YF
Tel: 01444 414290

Information; food and environmental allergies

British Society of Allergy and
Environmental Medicine
with the British Society of
Nutritional Medicine
PO Box 28
Totton
Southampton
SO40 2ZA

Mesotherapy

Dr Elisabeth Dancey
55 Wimpole Street
London
W1M 7DF
Tel: 0171 224 1330
Fax: 0171 486 1210

Dance

Imperial Society of Teachers of
Dancing
Euston Hall
Birkenhead Street
London
WC1H 8BE
Tel: 0171 837 9967
Fax: 0171 833 5981

Exercise

Both the RSA and YMCA provide excellent training for tuition of aerobics, step aerobics and other exercise classes. You should ensure that any class leader is qualified.

Ionothermie

Ionothermie Ltd
9–11 Alma Road
Windsor
Berkshire
SL4 3HU
Tel: 01753 833900
Fax: 01753 833553

NUTRITIONAL SUPPLEMENTS AND PUBLICATIONS

Lamberts Healthcare Ltd
1 Lamberts Road
Tunbridge Wells
Kent
TN2 3EQ
Tel: 01892 513116

MANUAL LYMPHATIC DRAINAGE

Manual Lymphatic Drainage
UK
8 Wittenham Lane
Dorchester on Thames
Oxon
OX10 7JW

OSTEOPATHY

Osteopaths can be found in Yellow Pages and should be members of the Register of Osteopaths (MRO).

CHIROPRACTIC

Chiropractors can be found in Yellow Pages and should be members of the British Chiropractic Association (BCA).

ALEXANDER TECHNIQUE, PILATES STUDIOS

Can be found in Yellow Pages.

INDEX